CORNEAL TRANSPLANTATION

An Immunological Guide to the Clinical Problem

CORNEAL TRANSPLANTATION

An Immunological Guide to the Clinical Problem

John V. Forrester
Lucia Kuffova
University of Aberdeen Medical School

ICP
Imperial College Press

Published by

Imperial College Press
57 Shelton Street
Covent Garden
London WC2H 9HE

Distributed by

World Scientific Publishing Co. Pte. Ltd.
5 Toh Tuck Link, Singapore 596224
USA office: Suite 202, 1060 Main Street, River Edge, NJ 07661
UK office: 57 Shelton Street, Covent Garden, London WC2H 9HE

British Library Cataloguing-in-Publication Data
A catalogue record for this book is available from the British Library.

CORNEAL TRANSPLANTATION: AN IMMUNOLOGICAL GUIDE TO THE CLINICAL PROBLEM

ISBN 1-86094-449-3

Printed by FuIsland Offset Printing (S) Pte Ltd, Singapore

For Thomas and Samuel

Contents

Preface

Corneal transplantation is the commonest type of solid tissue transplant, yet it remains in the realm of the esoteric both for the general ophthalmic surgeon, who rarely has the opportunity to perform this operation, and for the transplant surgeon, who regards the unusual immunological events going on in a corneal graft with some suspicion. Even for the transplant immunologist, the mechanism of rejection does not "obey the rules", as Wayne Streilein describes it. This book provides a summary of the various aspects of corneal transplantation—the clinical, immunological, therapeutic and prosthetic components—in one volume. The interested specialist in one field can thus have access to information from the other fields and develop a broad concept of the challenges to be faced in achieving the ultimate goal, i.e. an optically clear, visually satisfactory, functioning corneal graft which is tolerated in the long term without the need for systemic immunosuppression.

A second purpose of this book is to clear up certain misconceptions regarding corneal grafts. Corneal grafts have developed an enviable reputation for acceptance but this is true only for the first year or so and is probably due to the routine use of topical steroid therapy. When therapy is withdrawn graft rejection rates rise, induced by apparently trivial events such as removal of sutures. This is one example of innate immunity (minor trauma) driving adaptive immunity (graft rejection). On the other hand, it is still quite remarkable that without any form of tissue or blood group matching the one-year acceptance rate is so high. It is clear that acceptance rates for corneal grafts are not strictly comparable with other solid organ grafts. Despite this, the cornea has much to teach the transplant immunologist. Rejection for this tissue is almost exclusively by way of the indirect pathway and this process is gaining increasing importance in other types of graft rejection. In addition, the possible role of tissue antigens (effectively autoantigens) in the response to corneal allograft allows the clear dissection of these mechanisms in experimental models.

Acknowledgements. This book owes much to Martin Filipec, Head of the Department of Ophthalmology, Charles University, Prague, Czech Republic, not only for his encouragement in introducing the authors to this field but also for his collaborations through the years, for which we are truly grateful. In addition, we thank him for permission to use the clinical photographs taken by Lucie Stránská in Chapter 3. We would also like to thank Keryn Williams, of Flinders University, Australia, for providing us with photographs of corneal graft in sheep (Chapters 8 and 10), and May Griffith, of Laval University, Quebec, Canada, for her photographs of synthetic corneal grafts (Chapter 13). Heping Xu, of Aberdeen University, Scotland, kindly provided the image of the corneal endothelium for Figure 4.1C. We would like to thank also the audiovisual technical staff Stuart Duncan, Ian Harold and John Sangster and graphic artists and technical staff Gordon Stables and Daniel Eaton, from the Department of Medical Illustration, University of Aberdeen, for producing the cartoons, drawings and video clips included in this book. Finally, thanks are also due to the many collaborators and students who stimulated discussions which allowed the development of many of the arguments and concepts outlined in the book. They include Vladimír Holáň and collaborators in his laboratory, Andrew D. Dick, Zdenka Hašková, Jarmilla Plšková, Li Cai, Magdaléna Sosnová and Klára Sedláková. We also wish to acknowledge the financial support of the University of Aberdeen Development Trust and the Campaign for Saving Sight in Grampian.

Note Added. In the final stage of proofreading the manuscript, news came to us of the sudden and untimely death of Dr Wayne Streilein, President of the Schepens Eye Institute. His leading role and massive contribution to the knowledge of corneal immunology, and immunology in general, cannot be overstated and his absence from the field will be deeply felt.

1

A Brief History of Corneal Transplantation

Ancient History

The history of "tissue transplantation" starts from Adam and Eve in Eden. Throughout history, however, the eye, as the avenue to the Sun God, has symbolized virtue and wisdom, with blindness as a penalty for impiety and the stigma of sexual shame. Blind people were generally regarded as social outcasts, for whom treatment of any sort represented a tampering with God's proper judgment. In myths and folklore, although occasionally the damaged eye was replaced by the fresh one (as happened to St Lucy, and to the unfortunate army surgeon of Grimm's fairy tale whose feline transplant betrayed itself by constantly spotting mice), the eye is more usually replaced by its symbolic equivalent of wisdom or second sight.

The search for a treatment for corneal scarring goes back to ancient Egyptian times, when it was customary to attempt a cosmetic improvement by rubbing in "lampblack" or soot. During the Greek civilization, and especially at the time of Hippocrates (*c.* 1500 BC), when significant advances were made in medicine generally, the various parts of the eye were described in detail, yet there was no reference to corneal surface diseases or scars. In the early Roman period (*c.* 131–200 AD) the first ocular treatment was performed by Galen [1]. He tattooed corneal scars using copper sulphate reduced with nutgall to achieve a better cosmetic appearance.

The 18th and 19th Centuries

At this time ophthalmology was still submerged in general surgery and, as a consequence, fair game for quacks and charlatans. The concept of surgical intervention to help and improve the vision of people with opaque corneas began in the second half of the 18th century, when, in an early English reference, two techniques to treat damaged corneas were described. One was "to pare off the excrescence with a small curved knife leaving as few inequalities as possible" and the other was "to scrub the eye with small brush made of 'barley' bristles". In 1771 Frenchman Guillaume Pellier de Quengsy first suggested replacing opaque corneas with glass or other transparent material inside a silver ring that would be sutured to the sclera [2]. He provided details of the proposed technique and counselled that the patient should lie flat rather than sit upright as was usual for other surgical procedures on the eye at that time. He also wisely advised that patient should lie flat for a further eight days postoperatively, in case the implant fell out. However, he never performed this procedure either on humans or in experimental models. Later in 1775 Robert Mead advised a nonsurgical technique, in which equal parts of glass and sugar might be efficacious in improving vision due to the damaged cornea when rubbed into the eyes daily.

In time, ophthalmology emerged as a separate subspecialty of general surgery. In the wake of the French Revolution came the Napoleonic wars, with their legacy to the scores of soldiers and sailors blinded by the Egyptian Ophthalmia. For these conditions, new specialized "eye centres" for treatment of eye diseases were established in 19th century Europe (Moorfields, London, in 1805 and Royal Westminster, London, in 1816) and the United States (New London, 1817) and the notion of transplanting animal corneas to humans was gaining attention. Unfortunately the precise animal experiment could not been performed due to the lack of anaesthesia, sufficiently fine instruments and sutures, and an absence of antiseptic principles. There followed a period in which there was general disbelief that the excised cornea could in any case survive. This idea was dispelled in 1835 when, using a modified surgical technique, but with normal corneal tissue, Samuel Bigger reported the first successful corneal allograft, performed in this case in a pet gazelle [3]. This report kept interest in keratoplasty alive and in 1844 Kissam in New York reported that in 1838 he had transplanted a portion of young pig's cornea to the eye of a man blind from central leucoma [4]. This was the first attempt to transplant a xenograft into man but, being before its time, the underlying immunological principles were not appreciated, and in 1844 another report was published by Wutzer, who transplanted a sheep's cornea into a human being. In both cases the transplantation succeeded with good tissue healing and lack of panuveitis, but the corneas ultimately became opaque.

Perhaps due to the disappointing visual results with living tissue surgeons turned to artificial transplants. In 1853 Nussbaum tested gold, silver, copper and glass balls so he could determine the most inert substance for artificial corneas [5]. He had chosen glass and in later animal experiments he embedded 3 mm glass buttons into the cornea of the rabbits unfortunately with inevitable failure through infection.

However, with the development of finer instruments for ophthalmic surgery and the invention of the direct ophthalmoscope for investigation of patients, post surgical examinations showed the vast potential of ophthalmic surgery which could be offered to the world [6] and interest in corneal transplantation remained high.

Later experiments on animals performed by Power (1872) and Wolfe (1879) led to new conclusions regarding what could be achieved [7]. Firstly, it was clear that the cornea could maintain viability and transparency when transplanted from one site to another, but to be successful it must be taken from a freshly enucleated human eye; secondly, it was important that all incisions in the cornea were clean, that measurement of the graft was exact, and finally, that subjacent structures (conjunctival and scleral tissue) involved in keratoplasty must not be damaged.

By the end of the 19th century general anaesthesia was widely used to replace stupefaction by alcohol and opium, which had been the only analgesics used in earlier times. Ether and later chloroform were used in general surgery, and cocaine as local anaesthetic was used in 1884 by Koller and Schleich. In 1889 Schleich was responsible for the introduction of infiltration anaesthesia.

The outstanding experimental and clinical work of Arthur von Hippel towards the end of the 19th century showed that the corneal endothelium and Descemet's membrane must remain intact if a corneal graft was to succeed [8]. Thereafter, lamellar keratoplasty, in which partial thickness of the recipient cornea was removed, but full-thickness donor cornea was applied, together with a clockwork mechanical trephine, which replaced knives and cork borer, improved the outcome of corneal transplantation. Reports of von Hippel's success encouraged other surgeons to follow his technique and notable amongst these studies were thirty cases reported by Fuchs with eleven good results and improved vision in two full-thickness cases [9].

Thus, favourable conditions for the first successful human full-thickness keratoplasty were set up. General anaesthesia was in widespread use, surgical instruments had improved, and there was some degree of control of infection.

The Early 20th Century

At the beginning of the 20th century (1905 in Olomouc, Czech Republic) Edward Konrad Zirm for the first time successfully transplanted the cornea from a young male donor whose eye had been injured by a foreign body into a male patient who was blind following a lime burn [10–12]. This was the first case of a full-thickness graft, which was carefully investigated and followed up for 18 months with accurate observations of visual improvement during that period. Zirm modified von Hippel's technique by using overlay sutures and as a result he postulated principles for successful corneal transplantation. These were: strict use of human cornea from young and otherwise healthy individuals for the grafting procedure; use of Hippel's trephine together with adequate anaesthesia and asepsis during the surgical procedure and with adequate retention of the donor cornea by overlay sutures.

At the beginning of World War I, Elschnig became a protagonist of the full thickness corneal graft and his work influenced ophthalmic surgeons to move towards to full-thickness graft in same way as von Hippel's work towards lamellar grafts in previous century [13].

Consequently, modifications of Zirm's technique using overlay of the graft with different patterns of sutures, different shapes of graft and different methods for fixation (e.g. penetrating vs nonpenetrating sutures), and the use of the egg (yolk sac) membrane to secure the corneal graft, were published and performed by variety of surgeons. These included some of the most famous names in ophthalmology: Elschnig from the Prague school; Filatov from the Russian school; Castroviejo, Katzin, Maclean and Paton from the United States; Barraquer and Arruga from the Spanish school. In the middle of the 20th century co-operation among three French surgeons, Paufique, Sourdille and Offret, together with Swiss colleagues Franceschetti and others resulted in a landmark publication, "*Les Greffes de la Cornee*", in 1948 [14–17].

The Modern Era

The modern era of corneal transplantation started in the 1950s with improvements in surgical techniques and the development of very fine artificial sutures and instruments for corneal grafting and intraocular manipulation, a better understanding of the immunology and pathophysiology of corneal grafts, improved eye-banking methods and the use of anti-inflammatory drugs to control corneal graft rejection.

Even today, immunological rejection of the cornea is still the greatest limiting factor to successful corneal grafting and the distinction of its recognition as a clinical entity belongs to Edward Maumenee [18]. There followed a series of classic experiments, describing corneal graft rejection scientifically through the systematic study of the rabbit allograft model, elegantly designed by Khodadoust, whose name is linked with the endothelial rejection line, and Silverstein [19].

Townley Paton realized the constant need for the supply of viable corneal tissue, and founded the New York Eye Bank in 1959, which led to the setting up of the Eye Bank Association of America in 1961. The standards laid down by this organization have had considerable influence on the procurement, preservation, storage and use of donor tissue in the United States and throughout the world.

While on the one hand the surgical microscope has had an overwhelming impact on operative techniques, on the other side the specular microscope pointed out the importance of the healthy and functioning endothelium as a key to successful penetrating keratoplasty.

The history of corneal graft surgery would not be complete without mentioning the name of Sir Peter Medawar and his initial work on the immunology of skin grafts [20]. The discovery of acquired tolerance, which he described with Billingham and Brent, was probably his greatest achievement, for which he shared the Nobel Prize with Macfarlane Burnet in 1960. However, he also made numerous contributions to the study of graft rejection and he played an important role in demonstrating the activity of antilymphocyte serum and the mechanism of its action.

Many problems remain in controlling corneal graft rejection and in particular the success of corneal grafting is severely limited in particular types of corneal diseases such as vascularized corneal tissue, corneas after alkali burn and in eyes with surface healing problems. The extensive research in artificial corneas will bring further advances in corneal grafting in such "high risk" recipients. Also tissue engineering will help us overcome problems with limited numbers of corneal tissue donors in future (see Chapter 13). Increasing knowledge of the role specific cells play in corneal physiology, such as the much-vaunted limbal stem cell, help towards a combined or multistaged approach to managing "high risk" corneal grafts.

Even if the whole-eye transplant of popular fantasy and fable will not be possible for the foreseeable future, it is certain that with further advances in immunology and technology there will be hope for the vast reserve of potential patients in developed and less developed parts of the world and especially for patients with severely damaged corneas, who are, at the moment, left in a world of blindness.

References

1. Trevor-Roper PD. The history of corneal grafting. In: Casey TA, *Corneal Grafting.* Butterworths, London, 1972; 1.
2. De Quengsey P. *Precis au cours d'operations sur la chirgie des yeux.* Paris, *Didot*, 1789.
3. Bigger S. Inquiry into the possibility of transplanting the corneas, with the view of relieving blindness (hitherto deemed uncurable) caused by several diseases of that structure. *Dublin J Med Sci* 1837; 11: 408.
4. Kissam RS. *N Y J Med* 1844; 2: 281.
5. Nussbaum J. *Cornea Artificialis.* Munich, 1853.
6. Walton HH. Transplantation of the cornea. In: Walton HH, *Operative Ophthalmic Surgery.* Lindsay & Blakiston, Philadelphia, 1853; 379.
7. Power H. *IV International Congress of Ophthalmology*, Vol 4. London, 1872; 172.
8. Von Hippel A. *Albrecht v Graefes Arch Ophthal* 1888; 34: 108.
9. Wood CA. *The American Encyclopedia and Dictionary of Ophthalmology.* In Vol V, *Conjunctivitis-Dioptrics.* Chicago-Cleveland Press, 1914; 3483.
10. Zirm E. *Eine erfolgreich totale Keratoplastik. Arch Ophthalmol* 1906; 64: 580.
11. Snyder C. Alois Glogar, Karl Brauer and Eduard Konrad Zirm. *Arch Ophthalmol* 1965; 74(6): 871.
12. Fanta H. Eduard Zirm (1863–1944). *Klin Monatsbl Augenheilkd* 1986; 189(1): 64.
13. Casey TA and Mayer DJ. The history of corneal grafting. In *Corneal Grafting: Principles and Practice.* Saunders, Philadelphia, 1984; 9.
14. Mannis MJ and Krachmer JH. A historical perspective. *Surv Ophthalmol* 1981; 25: 333.
15. Rycroft BW. History. In: Rycroft BW, *Corneal Grafts.* Butterworth & Co, London, 1955; 1.
16. Castroviejo R. Corneal transplants or keratoplasty. In: Spaeth EB, *The Principles and Practice of Ophthalmic Surgery.* Lea & Febiger, Philadelphia, 1939; 470.
17. Forstat SL and Kaufman HE. Corneal transplantation. *Ann Rev Med* 1977; 28: 21.
18. Silverstein AM. Contributions of A. Edward Maumenee to ocular immunology. *Am J Ophthalmol* 1979; 88(3 Pt 1): 302.

19. Khodadoust AA and Silverstein AM. Local graft versus host reactions within the anterior chamber of the eye: the formation of corneal endothelial pocks. *Invest Ophthalmol* 1975; 14(9): 640.
20. Brent L. Fetally and neonatally induced immunologic tolerance. In *A History of Transplantation Immunology*. Academic Press, London, 1997; 227.

2

Surgery of Corneal Graft in Humans

Introduction

Keratoplasty or corneal transplantation is the operative replacement of damaged corneal tissue by healthy corneal tissue. The corneal graft may be lamellar (partial thickness of the grafted cornea) or penetrating (full thickness of the grafted cornea). The major goals of corneal transplantation are to improve vision, maintain the integrity of the globe and in some cases decrease pain. There are other surgical procedures such as photorefractive keratectomy, partial or total conjunctival flaps or artificial keratoprothesis, which can be used to achieve these goals. Therefore a careful consideration of suitable patients in the preoperative phase is important. The postoperative follow-up is crucial for all transplanted patients and penetrating keratoplasty is contraindicated in noncompliant patients or noncompliant parents of a child or infant requiring a corneal graft. In such cases even the best surgical result can become a greater problem than the original indication for which penetrating keratoplasty was performed.

Indications for Corneal Graft

The indications for penetrating keratoplasty are several.

Optical indications

Optical indications infer that improvement of visual acuity is the major aim for replacing an opaque cornea, or a clear but misshapen cornea, with clear donor tissue. Currently the most common optical indication is pseudophakic bullous keratopathy (major indication in the USA and UK), but there are others, such as keratoconus (major indication in the Czech Republic and Australia), corneal dystrophies and degenerations, and scarring caused by various types of infective and non-infective keratitis and trauma.

Tectonic indications

A tectonic graft is one where preservation and restoration of ocular anatomy is the major aim of surgery. Eyes with severe structural abnormalities of the cornea and anterior part of the eye such as imminent corneal thinning, corneal injury with the loss of tissue and large descemetocele are examples of this indication.

Therapeutic indications

Corneal graft may also be performed primarily for medical indications i.e. as a therapy. Such indications include removal of inflamed corneal tissue in eyes unresponsive to conventional antimicrobial, antiparasitic or antiviral therapy.

Cosmetic indications

Here the primary aim is to improve the appearance of the eye [1].

Surgical Factors Affecting Graft Outcome

During the last 20 years, there have been significant advances in the development of the technique of corneal transplantation and several factors have contributed towards this:

(1) Finer and better surgical materials, including both the extremely delicate needles and the very fine sutures, which induce less strong tissue reaction and reduce frequency of tissue necrosis. Previously, this local tissue response frequently led to the neovascularization on the cornea,

infiltration and ultimately rejection of the corneal graft and was a clear example of how an innate immune response to a foreign material (suture) contributed towards the initiation of the adaptive immune response (see Chapter 6).

In addition, improvements in instrumentation for corneal surgery have greatly affected outcomes. Delicate forceps, needle-holders, trephines, dissectors and special corneal scissors instead of the previously used knives are available now to perform corneal graft surgery. This minimizes tissue damage in both the donor and the recipient eye and subsequent loss of transparency of the corneal graft.

(2) Individual surgical skills and surgical technique. Large multicentre audits have confirmed that experienced corneal surgeons with high levels of surgical skills have a better track record of corneal graft survival.

(3) Preoperative and postoperative management. As previously mentioned careful choice of suitable candidates for corneal transplantation is crucial for a good final result after corneal transplantation. Regular follow-up and use of local and systemic anti-inflammatory and immunosuppressive medication especially for patients at "higher risk" of corneal graft rejection greatly improves corneal graft survival.

(4) Developments in corneal banking and advances in corneal preservation have also greatly improved outcomes in corneal transplantation (see Chapter 4). Use of specially prepared storage medium for corneal material has extended the time that corneal tissue can be preserved and augmented the viability of preserved tissue. This has led to improved tissue selection guidelines to meet increasing demand for high quality donor corneas (see Chapter 4).

Types of Corneal Graft

There are several types of corneal graft, each applied for a different set of indications.

Lamellar keratoplasty

The biggest expansion in corneal transplantation history came with the technique of lamellar keratoplasty towards the end of the 19th century [2, 3]. It was described first by von Hippel in 1877, who showed that it was possible to use a trephine to prepare a human donor corneal graft, which would be the same size and shape as the defect in the recipient cornea. In the initial description the corneal graft was not sutured, but was kept in place only by pressure of the eyelids. Eleven years later von Hippel presented his new technique of circumscribed lamellar keratoplasty where he replaced a partial thickness disc of the host's leucomatous cornea by a disc of the same diameter, but full-thickness, taken from the cornea of a dog. He also claimed that this technique was easier to perform than full-thickness keratoplasty and it was also less liable to loss of vitreous and displacement of other intraocular structures such as a lens. In his experiences, by the end of the third week the transplant was completely healed to the surrounding tissue of the host. Although the transplanted tissue and host cornea healed together by scar tissue, which never clarified completely, the vision after surgery was reported as improved.

Further modifications of the procedure for lamellar keratoplasty were published in 1908 by Plange, where he inserted oval full-thickness corneal grafts, like the face of a watch, into a corneal stromal pocket; and in 1910 by Löhlein, who used conjunctival flaps of the donor for securing a full-thickness corneal transplant. Morax in 1912 presented a method of keratoplasty by transposition; interchanging a transplant, obtained with a trephine from the periphery of the cornea, with a similar disc obtained in the opacified pupillary zone of the same eye [2–6].

Currently, three modifications of lamellar keratoplasty are widely used. In *inlay lamellar keratoplasty*, the anterior part (2/3) of the recipient corneal stroma is removed and replaced with partial thickness donor cornea (Figure 2.1). The major goal in inlay lamellar keratoplasty is to replace superficial abnormal corneal tissue or to add additional corneal tissue into the areas of the cornea to provide strength [7, 8]. The major indications for this procedure are peripheral corneal thinning, peripheral corneal perforations, pterygia and any corneal disorders, which involve only anterior layers of the cornea.

Deep lamellar keratoplasty is a subtype of inlay lamellar keratoplasty in which the entire corneal stroma is removed down to the Descemet's membrane [9–13]. The difference between deep lamellar keratoplasty and classic inlay lamellar keratoplasty is qualitative rather than quantitative. In the first technique, the anatomical properties of the cornea provide clear separation of the stroma and Descemet's membrane. This plane has a clear and smooth surface. On the contrary, classical *inlay lamellar keratoplasty* with dissection involving only the anterior 2/3 of the stroma results in a very rough and uneven surface with a risk of significant residual scarring and low visual acuity [14–16].

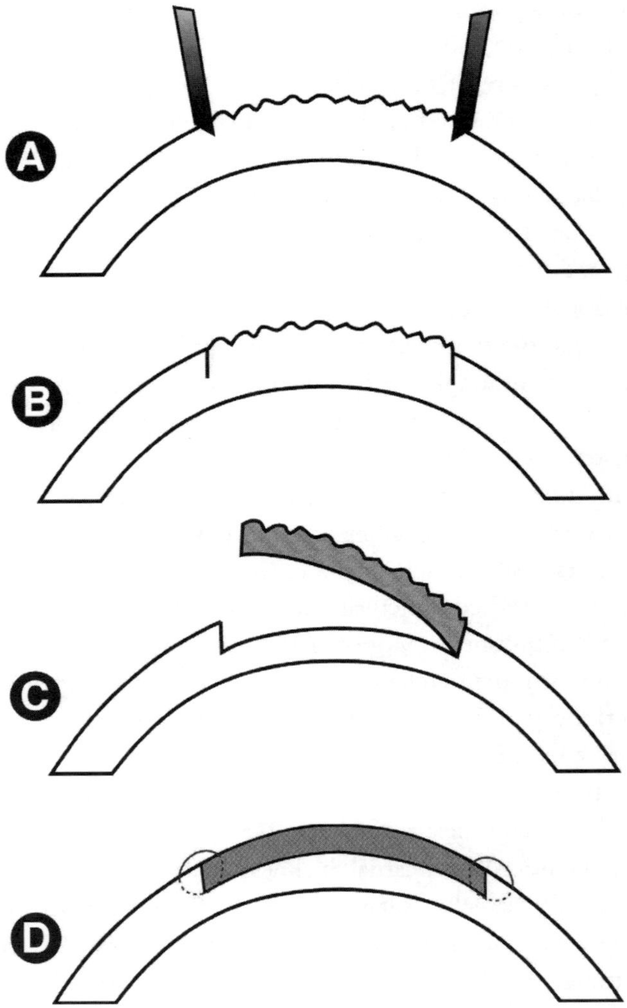

Figure 2.1 Inlay lamellar keratoplasty. (**A**) The first stage of the procedure involves keratectomy by trephination of the cornea. The size and position of the keratectomy and donor graft are variable and depend on the position of the lesions in the anterior corneal stroma. To treat keratoconus by inlay lamellar keratoplasty, the keratectomy bed should extend at least 0.5 mm beyond the edge of the cone. For necrotic, infective corneas or descemetoceles, the keratectomy bed should include the entire area plus a rim of healthy tissue. (**B**) Trephination is partial thickness (0.2–0.3 mm depth) and lamellar dissection of the abnormal corneal epithelium and anterior stroma is performed either by peeling or with dissecting instrument. (**C**) The lamellar flap is held with forceps and either steadily peeled manually from periphery to the centre of the diseased cornea or is dissected with a cyclodialysis spatula, surgical knife or stainless blade. With a similar technique the donor lamellar graft is prepared either from fresh intact eye or from preserved lyophilized tissue. (**D**) The donor lamellar graft is secured into the keratoplasty bed with a running suture or interrupted sutures.

In *onlay lamellar keratoplasty* a partial thickness donor cornea is placed on de-epithelized cornea in which a small peripheral keratectomy and/or peripheral lamellar dissection has been done (Figure 2.2). The main aim in onlay lamellar keratoplasty is reinforcing of thin, ectatic corneas in patients with keratokonus, keratoglobus, or corneal pellucid marginal degeneration [17].

The major advantages of onlay and inlay lamellar keratoplasty are: both procedures avoid the risk of serious vision-threatening complications or permanent vision loss which can be associated with any intraocular procedure; an onlay lamellar keratoplasty is removable, which permits penetrating full-thickness keratoplasty to be performed later, if previous surgery was not successful; and the risk of graft rejection in onlay lamellar keratoplasty is minimal [17].

The advantages of onlay lamellar keratoplasty over inlay lamellar keratoplasty are: the preparation of recipient bed is technically less demanding and less time-consuming; risk of corneal perforation is minimal and the procedure is reversible. The disadvantages of inlay lamellar keratoplasty include reduced visual acuity as a result of interface irregularities caused by uneven lamellar dissection of the recipient, and in some cases of the donor tissue, opacities in the donor–recipient interface, and higher risk of graft rejection compared to onlay lamellar keratoplasty.

Unlike full-thickness penetrating keratoplasty and posterior lamellar keratoplasty lamellar/onlay and inlay/keratoplasty do not require fresh corneal donor tissue.

Posterior lamellar keratoplasty is the latest modification of lamellar keratoplasty (Figure 2.3). In this modification the posterior stroma and the diseased corneal endothelium are removed [10, 18, 19]. The major indications are Fuchs' endothelial dystrophy and pseudophakic bullous keratopathy. In this case the corneal surface of the recipient and also anterior corneal stroma is left intact and the donor posterior stromal lamellae together with endothelial donor tissue are introduced through a limbal scleral incision. The graft is stabilized in the prepared graft bed with a bubble of air, which is injected into the anterior chamber of the eye of the graft recipient at the end of the operation. Postoperatively, the surface corneal topography remains smooth without any significant change in astigmatism. Early experiences with this technique have shown predictable corneal power with healthy corneal endothelium and better corneal endothelial cell counts than those occurring after full-thickness penetrating keratoplasty [18]. The primary challenge in this procedure is to achieve consistent interface smoothness and optical clarity along the recipient and donor resection with consistent depth of the corneal tissue.

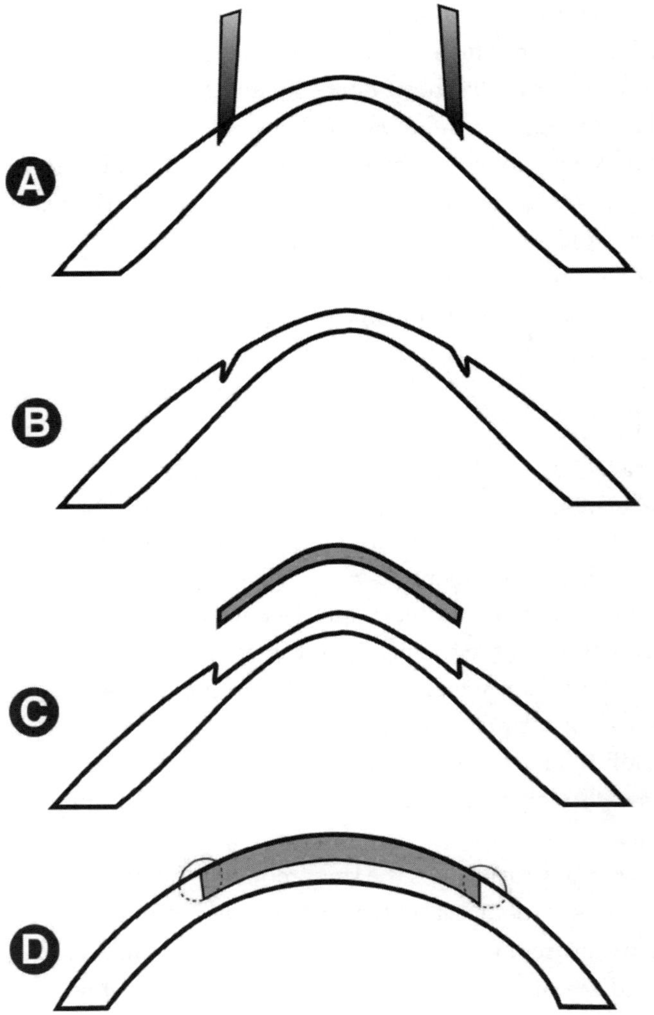

Figure 2.2 Onlay lamellar keratoplasty. (**A**) The central epithelium is removed with a Paton spatula. The peripheral epithelium at the limbus is left intact to aid and enhance the speed of re-epithelization. A Barron vacuum trephine is placed on the cornea in such a way that the cone is surrounded with the blade. (**B**) A partial thickness cut is made into the healthy cornea with a vacuum trephine and this procedure is followed by preparing a circumferential 0.5-mm-wide wedge with Vannas scissors. The result is an annular keratectomy 0.5 mm wide where the deepest part is nearest to the limbus. The prepared donor lamellar graft is carefully rinsed and inspected for any possible debris. (**C**) The donor tissue is attached to the recipient bed with 16 interrupted 10-0 nylon sutures. (**D**) A Paton spatula is used to flatten the ectatic corneal tissue as interrupted sutures are evenly sutured into place. Immediately after surgery multiple folds are visible under the corneal graft as the original tissue was compressed and flattened during the surgery. These usually disappear within six weeks after surgery.

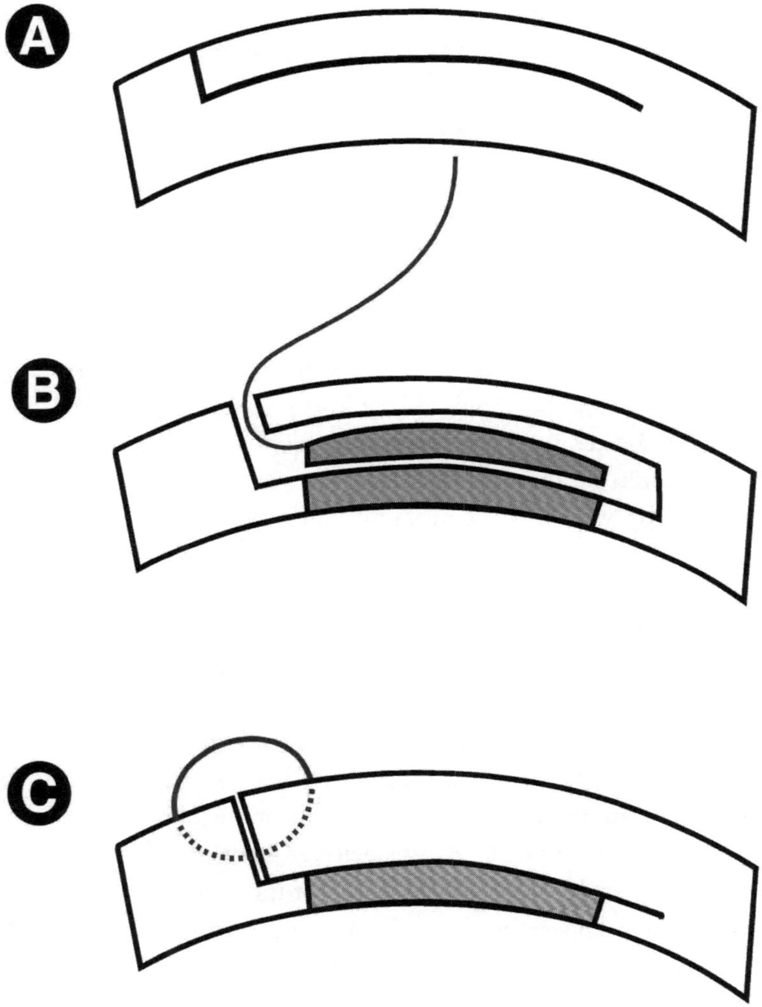

Figure 2.3 Posterior lamellar keratoplasty. (**A**) A limbal incision measuring about 9 mm in diameter is made in the sclera extending to about one-third of the scleral depth. (**B**) A deep lamellar intrastromal pocket is then prepared extending from one side of the limbus to the other into which is placed a customised intrastromal trephine. A 7.0–8.5 mm circular ring is cut into the anterior chamber. The posterior portion of the cornea, which includes the diseased endothelium and a portion of the posterior stroma, is then removed through the pocket wound. The donor tissue is prepared by mounting the corneoscleral cap onto an artificial chamber. A Barron Recipient Suction trephine is used on the surface to resect the anterior two-thirds of the corneal tissue. The donor tissue is placed endothelial side up on a standard punch block to obtain a posterior lenticule of the same diameter as the recipient resection. The lenticule is placed endothelial side down onto a spatula coated with viscoelastic material and placed into the anterior chamber, which has been filled with air. The spatula is lifted anteriorly and removed. (**C**) Air is placed into the anterior chamber to stabilize the graft and the superior scleral wound is closed with nylon sutures.

The disadvantages of posterior lamellar keratoplasty are: the technique is time-consuming, special instruments and a fresh donor cornea are required, the surgery as for any intraocular procedure, is vision threatening, but the main advantage is that the graft can be replaced if it is not successful, by penetrating keratoplasty.

Full-thickness penetrating keratoplasty

Development of full-thickness keratoplasty techniques

As mentioned before, the first successful human penetrating keratoplasty was performed in the beginning of the 20th century (Figure 2.4). In 1905 Eduard Zirm bilaterally transplanted corneas to a patient who sustained alkali burn while cleaning his chicken coop with lime. The donor was an 11-year-old boy who had a perforating injury of his eye, which required enucleation. Two grafts were retrieved from the single donor eye and recipient underwent bilateral keratoplasty. Remarkably, one of the grafts remained clear for several years.

This experience induced other eye surgeons to embark on the technique of full-thickness corneal transplantation. The first large series of 180 patients transplanted with human corneal homografts was reported by A. Elschnig in Prague. His data formed the basis for a set of protocols in which the indications, techniques and complications of penetrating keratoplasty were established [4, 20]. As was believed at the time, the ultimate fate of the graft depended more on the nature of the surrounding tissue of the host than on the appearance of the graft during the first few days. If the transplant was surrounded by a dense corneal leucoma, which was thought to greatly impair the nutrition of the graft, the transplanted tissue usually became cloudy or completely opaque. Another observation was that excessive bevelling during the preparation of the donor graft led to a greater tendency for the graft to protrude, and finally, when two separate sutures were used to hold graft in the position, occasionally one of the sutures had a tendency to indent the transplant more that the other. The developing lines of uneven pressure led to uneven coadaptation of the edges of the transplant and cornea of the host.

In the original technique the donor corneal graft was prepared by trephination of the freshly enucleated human eye and the maximum diameter for the donor corneal button was 4 mm. If a larger piece was trephined from the damaged host cornea, the transplanted donor corneal tissue could not be held in position by the temporarily placed conjunctival flap, and therefore

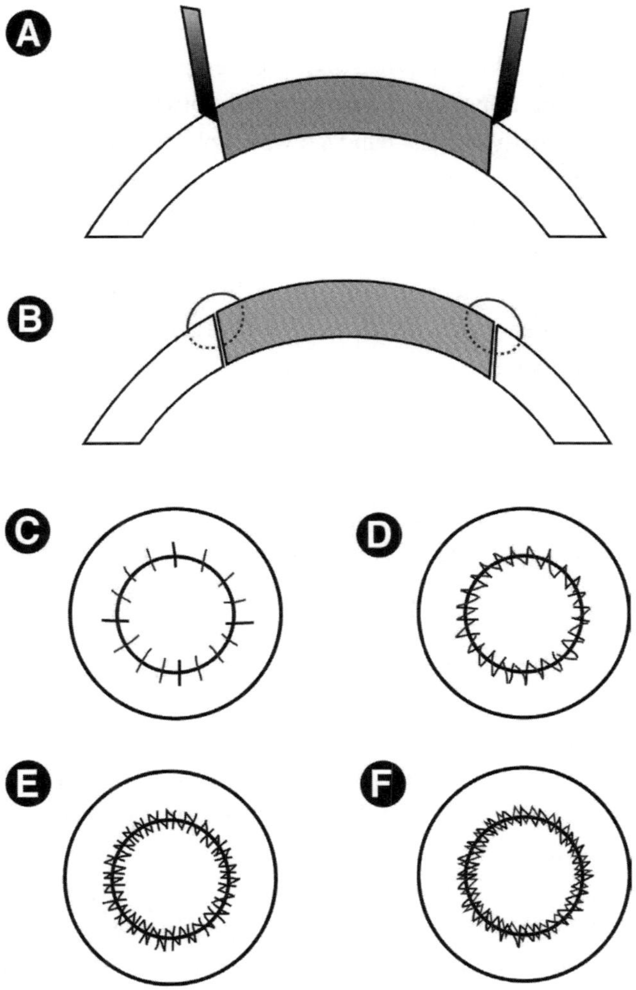

Figure 2.4 Full-thickness penetrating keratoplasty. (**A**) The size of the graft varies from 7.5 mm for males and 6.5–7 mm for females. The centre of the diseased cornea is measured and stained with a marker pen. A Barron vacuum trephine is placed exactly above the mark on the cornea and is attached with suction to the corneal surface and blade rotated to cut into the corneal tissue. The incision penetrates the full depth of the corneal stroma without entering the anterior chamber. The chamber is finally entered by incising through Descemets' membrane and completing the incision with curved corneal scissors after the anterior chamber is re-formed and deepened with viscoelastic material. The corneal button is finally removed and the donor button is placed orthotopically into the graft bed. The donor button is usually larger than original excised cornea (0.25 mm for phakic and pseudophakic eyes and 0.5 mm for aphakic eyes). (**B**) The donor cornea is fixed with four cardinal sutures at 12, 6, 3 and 9 o'clock and then additional interrupted or continuous sutures are placed into the stroma of the cornea. To secure the donor corneal graft in the recipient bed, various combinations of interrupted and continuous sutures are used: (**C**) interrupted suture 16-bites (10-0 nylon); (**D**) single running suture 24-bites (10-0 nylon); (**E**) combined interrupted (10-0 nylon) and single running (11-0 nylon) sutures; (**F**) combined double running (10-0 nylon) and (11-0 nylon) sutures.

the larger wound dehiscence had to be covered with conjunctival tissue. Postoperatively, the upper eye lid was carefully placed over the transplanted cornea and conjunctival flap, a bandage was applied to both eyes, which was kept in place for two days and the patient was confined to bed [4].

Before the introduction of specially designed corneal trephines, a corneal punch was used to excise the damaged and opaque corneal tissue from the host. This led to several technical problems. In the case of anterior synechie, which had not been separated by previous surgery at the time of corneal grafting, the iris tissue required careful separation and excision.

When retention sutures were used, these were properly adjusted so that they lay uniformly taut with slight pressure over the corneal graft. There were many modifications of placement of the retention sutures (Figure 2.5) [4, 20]. They were usually placed on the host cornea before trephination, so special attention had to be paid to ensure that the integrity of the sutures remained intact. To avoid additional damage to the grafted corneal epithelial layer by corneal sutures, the vitelline membrane of a boiled egg was placed over the corneal graft before tying them. If a conjunctival flap only was used to cover the graft, sutures were removed 10–12 days postsurgery and the flap was retracted or excised from the eye. If retention sutures were used, they were released and removed 12–14 days postsurgery. The postoperative complications, such as faulty position of the corneal graft, elevation of the intraocular pressure, damage to the lens at the time of trephination, prolapse of iris and/or vitreous tissue into the wound and leaky anterior chamber with formation of the anterior synechiae and finally endophthalmitis, were unfortunately not unusual complications after any type of intraocular surgery at this time.

Introduction of the corneal trephine and preparation of circular corneal discs for transplantation transformed the technique of corneal grafting and the trephine soon became an essential instrument. The trephine had to be placed perfectly vertically on the cornea, a guidemark on epithelium was made initially to check position of the trephine, and thereafter trephining was carried out with a steady and equal rotary movement. The essential point of this part of the surgery was to keep the anterior chamber of the eye intact and protect the iris and lens from further damage with trephine. The incision was completed with a small blade and curved scissors. Donor corneal graft was pre-prepared using a similar trephine and kept in a Petri dish. The graft was secured with edge-to-edge interrupted sutures, which did not enter the anterior chamber of the host and remained unrotated on the surface of the recipient cornea (Figure 2.6).

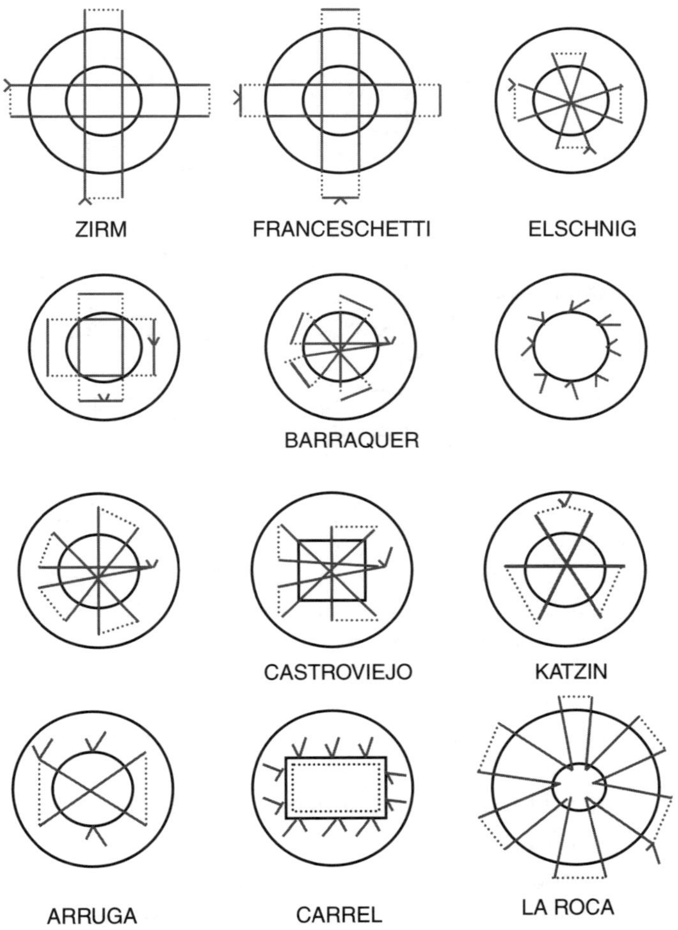

Figure 2.5 Different modifications of retention-bridge sutures and interrupted sutures. Retention-bridge sutures are placed into the recipient cornea before trephination of the diseased cornea and left in place for 10–14 days. (Dotted line represents the intrastromal placement of the suture; full line represents the position of the suture above the corneal epithelium. In the case of the Carrel modification the interrupted line indicates the inner part of the step position of the donor corneal graft.)

Another refinement of the technique—the step graft—initiated by Carrel, Eberling and Apolonio allowed more perfect closure of the anterior chamber (see Ref. 4). Its aim was to diminish postoperative complications and, above all, the refraction defects brought by ectasia and small gaps. Again the critical instrument for this kind of surgery was the trephine with an external guide, strictly concentric with it, and of the same diameter as the

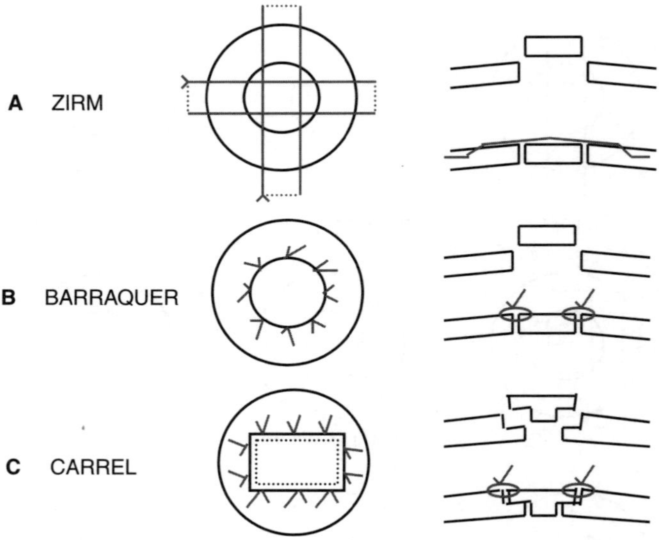

Figure 2.6 Various modifications of the position of the donor corneal graft in the recipient corneal bed. (**A**) Zirm modification—donor corneal graft placed into the recipient corneal bed edge-to-edge and secured with retention-bridge suture; (**B**) Barraquer modification—donor corneal graft placed into recipient corneal bed edge-to-edge and secured with interrupted suture; (**C**) Carrel modification—donor corneal graft placed into recipient corneal bed by step approach and secured with interrupted sutures.

trephine used for cutting the anterior layers. The difference between two trephines was 1–1.5 mm.

Catroviejo introduced a rectangular graft which needed a special knife with two parallel blades of variable distance [4]. The resection was initiated on its superior part and once the anterior chamber was entered, the dissection was continued with straight scissors. The graft was placed into the recipient bed and secured with edge-to-edge interrupted sutures. This graft, however, did not gain much popularity.

The use of interrupted sutures at this time was not the standard method to fix the corneal graft into the graft bed. Bridge-retention sutures were more common and successful in securing the graft, which was grossly dependent on establishing a uniform suture pressure across the surface of the graft. This pressure had to be sufficiently strong to ensure a watertight connection between corneal graft and bed of the graft. To avoid further damage of corneal epithelium by overlay threads, the vitelline membrane of boiled egg (Paufique), or a piece of fine gum-elastic cut with a trephine of slightly larger dimensions than the trephined area of the cornea was used, and placed between the corneal graft and overlayed sutures. Such membranes not only protected the corneal graft surface but also helped to distribute the pressure of the sutures more uniformly.

Current techniques

The major indications for performing full-thickness penetrating keratoplasty have gradually changed over the last 25 years. At the moment the most common indications are: aphakic or pseudophakic bullous keratopathy, opaque (previously rejected) corneal grafts, keratoconus, Fuchs' endothelial dystrophy, other corneal dystrophies, scarring or active keratitis secondary to virus, scarring with or without chronic inflammation, acute or chronic ulcerative conditions, trauma, interstitial keratitis, chemical burns, degenerations and congenital opacities [21].

The most common instrument for donor corneal button and recipient bed preparation is the vacuum or rotation trephine. A new technique, which is currently under investigation, for preparation of the donor graft and recipient bed is the excimer-laser-based trephine system [15]. The major advantage of this technique is the smooth cut and edges of the donor tissue, which are parallel with the recipient bed.

The donor tissue is stabilized in the recipient graft bed with various combinations of the sutures (Figure 2.4C–F). The most common combination is the use of 16 interrupted sutures since this allows for the possibility of removing sutures independently and according to the clinical need, e.g. for optical purposes such as astigmatism, or for suture-related complications. The sutures are placed into 2/3 depth of the corneal stroma [21]. The same depth of placement is applied to the modified continuous single or double running sutures techniques used by some surgeons for corneal grafting. Sutures are usually removed one year postcorneal transplantation, if there is no suture-related problem such as corneal neovascularization, suture-related infiltrate, infection, immune rejection, loosening of the suture or very high astigmatism.

A recently published new suturing technique is the deep suturing technique which consists either of a 16-bite 10-0 nylon running suture or 8 interrupted 10-0 nylon cross sutures placed into the mid-stroma of the cornea and exited through endothelium of recipient and donor. A running continuous suture is also placed superficially to secure the corneal wound [22]. This superficial suture is removed 3–4 months after surgery and the deep-placed sutures are left in place. This technique allows the patient an early postoperative visual rehabilitation, but there are some unanswered questions concerning endothelial cell damage during the surgery and the stability of the postoperative refraction.

Complications of Corneal Graft Surgery

Despite significant advances in microsurgery, corneal banking and surgical skills together with an extensive worldwide experience in corneal graft surgery, some serious vision-threatening, but in some cases preventable, complications can occur. It is very important to recognize and adequately treat such problems. The complications can be categorized as:

(1) Intraoperative complication: suprachoroidal haemorrhage;
(2) Early postoperative complications: persisting epithelial defect, keratitis, endophthalmitis, wound leak, iris incarceration with anterior synechiae formation, hyphema, high or low intraocular pressure and primary corneal graft failure;
(3) Late postoperative complications: microbial keratitis, infectious crystalline keratopathy, recurrence of or *de novo* herpetic keratitis, low-grade endophalmitis, suture-related keratitis, wound dehiscence, stripped Descemet's membrane, epithelial ingrowth, stromal ingrowth, retrocorneal fibrous membrane, glaucoma, persistent mydriasis, cataract, retinal detachment, macular edema, phototoxic macular damage, corneal graft rejection, recurrence of recipient corneal disease in grafts, astigmatism and transmission of donor disease (see Chapter 12).

Some of the mainly late postoperative complications are discussed in following chapters.

Combined Surgical Procedures

Many eyes with opaque cornea have multiple abnormalities, including cataract, glaucoma, surface ocular disease and vitreoretinal pathology. Corneal graft surgery is sometimes combined with other procedures to deal with these problems.

Full-thickness penetrating keratoplasty and cataract extraction

The coexistence of cataract and corneal disease is not uncommon. Early cataract will progress after penetrating keratoplasty surgery and the likelihood of cataract formation increases significantly after the age of 50 regardless of indication for corneal graft [23]. In patients after multiple corneal graft procedures where multiple local steroid drops or systemic steroids and immunosuppressive treatment are used, the likelihood of cataract formation is also very high. It is not uncommon that the condition of the cornea does not allow the visualization of the entire lens and therefore cataract surgery prior to corneal grafting is risky. On the other hand, cataract surgery after corneal grafting can damage the graft and subjects the patient to two separate operations, increases cost and delays visual rehabilitation. Accordingly, combined cataract and corneal graft surgery is frequently the operation of choice when faced with these decisions.

The triple procedure of penetrating keratoplasty, extracapsular cataract extraction and posterior chamber intraocular lens implantation, seems to have no significant worsening of outcome and refractive status in patients with Fuchs' endothelial dystrophy compared to two separate procedures [24]. Therefore this procedure may be a good compromise for patients with corneal opacity and incipient or mature cataract.

Although some surgeons advocate closed phacoemulsification for cataract surgery followed by penetrating keratoplasty [25], the most common approach is open sky extracapsular extraction through the recipient corneal opening. For dislocated or subluxated lenses the preferable technique is an intracapsular cataract extraction with a cryoprobe.

The position of the intraocular lens may be variable and depends on the condition of the eye behind the opaque cornea. It is preferable to implant an intraocular lens into the physiological position of original lens, i.e. into the lens capsular bag. However, in cases where the disruption to the anterior segment is such that there is a significant capsular tear, or after intracapsular cataract extraction in cases of dislocated lens, this is impossible. An alternative approach is to place a transscleral fixated intraocular lens (in the iridocilliary sulcus), an iris-fixated intraocular lens or an anterior chamber intraocular lens can be used. However, in the latter two cases there is considerable risk to the donor endothelium and, in these circumstances, visual rehabilitation using an aphakic contact lens may be a better option [21].

Full-thickness penetrating keratoplasty in the aphakic eye

In this instance, combined surgery involves penetrating keratoplasty with surgery to the vitreous gel. The most important step is core vitrectomy, which has to be done at the time of corneal grafting, otherwise the corneal graft has minimal chance of survival, since vitreocorneal contact is highly risky for endothelial cell viability [1, 6]. Following a deep anterior vitrectomy particular attention should be paid to any vitreous strands, which may be in contact with corneal endothelium postoperatively. The vitrectomy should be sufficient enough that if posterior vitreous detachment occurs postoperatively, vitreous will not prolapse into the anterior chamber, especially if there is no intraocular lens implantation. The procedure can be completed through the keratoplasty opening using an open-sky approach. Depending on the surgical conditions and potential complications, the surgeon may decide to implant an intraocular lens as part of the procedure. If there is sufficient posterior capsule to permit, a posterior chamber intraocular lens may be used, otherwise a transscleral fixated intraocular lens, an iris-fixated intraocular lens or an anterior chamber intraocular lens may be inserted as above.

There is rarely an indication to perform combined corneal graft, lensectomy and posterior vitrectomy for instance in a patient with severe long-standing congenital corneal opacities with cataract who has developed a retinal detachment with a large posterior retinal tear. Under these circumstances, it is possible to prepare a three-port posterior vitrectomy, perform the corneal trephination and lensectomy and using a temporary Aachen style keratoprosthesis (see Chapter 13) complete the posterior vitrectomy and retinal detachment repair before inserting the lens implant and finally suturing the corneal graft in place. Fortunately, the indications for such surgery are not frequent and the combined skills of the cornea and vitreous surgeon are rarely called upon.

Full-thickness penetrating keratoplasty in pseudophakic eyes

Currently pseudophakic bullous keratoplasty is one of the main indications for penetrating keratoplasty. The important decision here is whether to retain the original intraocular lens or replace it with a different type and/or different position of intraocular lens. Removal of an intraocular lens, which is easy to rotate, is relatively straightforward through an open-sky approach, lifting it into the anterior chamber and then removing it from the eye. Removal of an intraocular lens which is fixed in the eye, usually in the sulcus with fibrovascular tissue, can be difficult and may not be possible. In this circumstance, cutting of the haptics peripherally and removing only the optical part of the intraocular lens may be the best option. Haptics left in their original position will cause less damage to the delicate tissue of the iris and ciliary body than to attempt to remove them from the lens capsule, which may cause posterior capsule rupture with consequent vitreous loss, massive bleeding, and damage of the cilliary body or retina with later retinal detachment [21]. After removal of the intraocular lens, the decision to insert a second intraocular lens which may be more suitable for the patient, depends on the overall condition of the eye and whether the new lens can be placed into the posterior chamber, the original capsular bag, the iridociliary sulcus, fixated through iridocilliary sulcus or onto the iris, or finally placed in the anterior chamber.

Full-thickness penetrating keratoplasty in eyes with ocular surface disease: combined limbal stem cell transplantation

One of the main reasons for failure of corneal grafts is recurrent epithelial breakdown and persistent corneal defects. This sets up a chronic nonspecific (innate immune) inflammatory response which eventually induces graft rejection and failure. A major underlying problem is limbal "stem cell" deficiency in the host, for instance in patients in whom the original indication for graft was severe chemical burns or ocular pemphigoid. In the case of limbal deficiency and repetitive epithelial corneal defects the transplant inevitably leads to failure. A number of surgical procedures have been proposed to replace the corneal epithelium and therefore improve the ocular surface condition and the likelihood of corneal graft survival. These procedures can be performed either before actual corneal translantation takes place or at the same time as corneal transplantation.

Conjunctival autografts are useful in the case of unilateral disease. Four conjunctival grafts are retrieved from the healthy eye and transplanted into the limbal area of the affected eye, prepared by removal of superficial vascularized scar tissue. The grafts are anchored at the limbal area with interrupted sutures to the cornea. It is possible for the conjunctival epithelium to proliferate over the cornea but it does not acquire the properties of the corneal epithelium.

A more satisfactory approach is to use *limbal autografts*. The limbal autograft is also a technique which can be used for patients with unilateral disease. Two grafts at four clock-hour sectors are removed from the unaffected eye and sutured onto the cornea and denuded sclera [26, 27].

Epithelial allografts (keratoepithelioplasty), as originally described by Thoft, is another technique in which small corneal lenticules consisting of epithelium and thin slices of anterior stroma from the donor eye are transplanted to the host eye bed which has been prepared with a 360° conjunctival peritomy [28].

Limbal transplantation is currently the most common type of the surgery for replacement of damaged or absent corneal epithelial cells [29–31]. Surgeons usually take the donor limbal area together with small rims of corneal and conjunctival tissue (Figure 2.7). On the recipient cornea a peripheral lamellar excision of the original limbal area is prepared and the donor limbal graft can be inlaid into the corneoscleral bed. In the case of unilateral disease the surgeon can use an autograft, from the unaffected eye, but there is a limitation to the size of the graft. No more than 180° of limbus can be taken from the contralateral eye without causing limbal deficiency. In cases of bilateral disease allografting is necessary. The success of this type of heroic surgery is limited but, in appropriate cases, combined corneal transplantation together with limbal transplantation in eyes with severe ocular disorders can result in ambulatory vision for affected patients which is extremely gratifying and useful to the patient. Unfortunately a progressive decline of the visual outcome and graft survival is often unavoidable despite treatment with systemic immunosuppression.

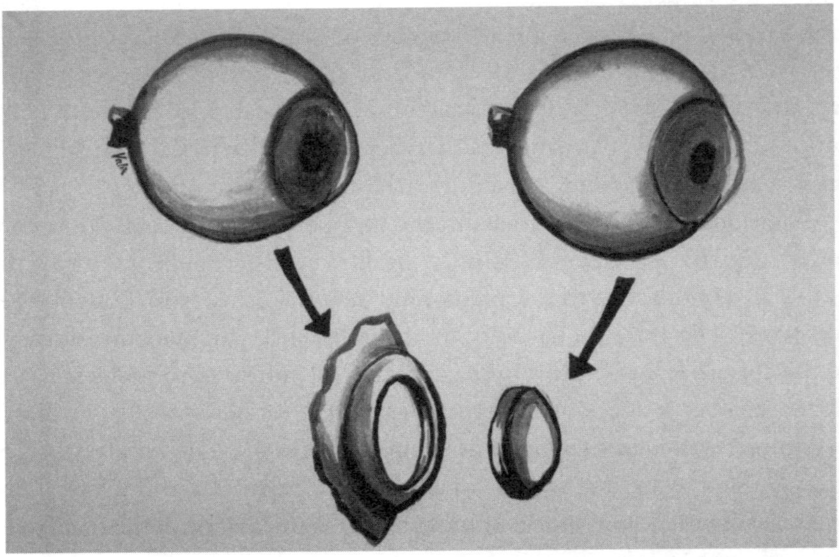

Figure 2.7 Combined penetrating corneal allotransplantation and limbal allografting. Two donor eyes (preferably from the same donor) are retrieved. The first eye is used as a source of donor full-thickness corneal graft and the second eye as a source of the donor limbal graft. The penetrating keratoplasty is performed in the usual manner, fixed with interrupted corneal sutures. The limbal allograft is inlayed in to the prepared sclerocorneal bed and secured with 10-0 nylon interrupted sutures in 360°.

Another approach, which can improve the quality of the ocular surface and prepare better conditions for corneal graft survival, is the use of cultured corneal stem cells on amniotic membranes [32–34]. In experiments on animals, it has been shown that after allotransplantation of corneal limbal stem cells with amnionic membranes, the ocular surface conditions improved. The ocular inflammation resolved, the cornea re-epithelialized, the stromal opacity declined, the superficial neovascularity was lessened and the conjunctival fornix re-established.

Full-thickness penetrating keratoplasty with corneoscleral graft

End stage corneal disease, such as occurs in eyes with extensive recurrent infections and epithelial downgrowth, has been treated in the past by anterior segment reconstruction using large corneoscleral grafts [35]. Common features of the surgical technique included a total limbal peritomy, use of oversized trephines (11–14 mm), and entry to the anterior chamber obliquely with a diamond knife leaving a ledge of sclera. The entire cornea is removed and in cases involving the iris and lens with epithelial downgrowth these structures are also removed .Although this technique can salvage an otherwise end stage eye, the results are poor with respect to maintenance of vision. The three major problems are recurrence of the original disease, glaucoma and graft rejection, the last of which inevitably leads to the loss of vision and ultimately to the loss of the eye. Glaucoma as a frequent complication can be controlled with topical medication or with a Molteno tube. Typical corneal rejection episodes are not common in eyes which survived the initial three weeks after grafting. However, atypical corneal rejection may explain the common occurrence of progressive corneal oedema. Another, probably more serious problem seems to be the recurrent and persistent nature of epithelial defects. This might also be explained by rejection of donor epithelium and a lack of host limbal stem cells. A prophylactic tarsorrhaphy appears to prevent the breakdown of the corneal epithelium and helps to rehabilitate the ocular surface.

This technique can be recommended only for patients with end stage eye disease, who have to be prepared for the likelihood of a poor visual outcome and the requirement of a regular, intensive follow-up.

Full-thickness penetrating keratoplasty with the corneal suture ring

Several modifications of full penetrating graft surgery have been devised to avoid astigmatism. One of these is the corneal suture ring. This is made of a cobalt titanium molybdenum alloy and is designed for suturing to the upper third of the undersurface of the wound to prevent corneal distortions resulting from pulled-through sutures [36, 37]. The corneal suture ring appears to accelerate healing and prevent immunological reactions in full-thickness penetrating keratoplasty. Unfortunately this device appears to have little influence on postoperative astigmatism. According to the inventor the ring also allows rapid epithelization and wound healing. As a result, sutures may be removed where necessary as early as three months postoperatively. And the rapid healing prevents deformation of the transplant and provides refractive stability in the early postoperative period. At the moment this technique is undergoing clinical trials, the results of which are not yet available. This surgical technique can be used in patients with favourable and also unfavourable prognosis of corneal graft survival.

Conclusion

The history of corneal graft surgery demonstrates the value of good clinical observations in guiding surgeons to an understanding of the immunopathological mechanisms and to developing new and better ways to prevent surgical complications, and to master the process of rejection. One of the most important considerations is good surgical technique and some clinical examples of different types of corneal grafts are shown in Chapter 3.

Unfortunately there remain many problems, not only with developing better ways to overcome chronic rejection but more immediately to understand, and deal with, many ocular surface problems. These are some of the challenges of today.

References

1. Coster DJ. Corneal transplantation. In: Coster DJ, *Cornea.* BMJ Books, 2002; BMJ Publishing Group, London, 2002; 128.
2. Meller J. Corneal transplantation. In: Meller J, *Ophthalmic Surgery.* Blakiston, New York, Toronto, 1912; 246.
3. Török E and Grout GH. Keratoplasty. In: Török E and Grout GH, *Surgery of the Eye.* Lea & Febiger, Philadelphia, New York, 1913; 136.
4. Castroviejo R. Corneal transplants or keratoplasty. In: Spaeth EB, *The Principles and Practice of Ophthalmic Surgery.* Lea & Febiger, Philadelphia, 1939; 470.
5. Meller J. Keratoplasty. In: Meller J, *Ophthalmic Surgery: A Handbook of Surgical Operations on Eyeball and Its Appendages.* Blakiston, New York, Toronto, 1952; 392.

6. Meyer W. Operations on the cornea. In: Meyer W, *Surgery of the Eye*. Grunde and Stratton, New York, 1949; 151.
7. Paufique L. Lamellar keratoplasty. In: Rycroft BW, *Corneal Grafts*. Butterworth & Co, London, 1955; 112.
8. Terry MA. The evolution of lamellar grafting techniques over twenty-five years. *Cornea* 2000; 19(5): 611.
9. Anwar M and Teichmann KD. Deep lamellar keratoplasty: surgical techniques for anterior lamellar keratoplasty with and without baring of Descemet's membrane. *Cornea* 2002; 21(4): 374.
10. Jain S and Azar DT. New lamellar keratoplasty techniques: posterior keratoplasty and deep lamellar keratoplasty. *Curr Opin Ophthalmol* 2001; 12(4): 262.
11. Trimarchi F, Poppi E and Klersy C. Deep lamellar keratoplasty. *J Fr Ophthalmol* 2002; 25(7): 718.
12. Sugita J and Kondo J. Deep lamellar keratoplasty with complete removal of pathological stroma for vision improvement. *Br J Ophthalmol* 1997; 81(3): 184.
13. Krumeich JH and Daniel J. Live epikeratophakia and deep lamellar keratoplasty for I-III stage-specific surgical treatment of keratokonus. *Klin Monatsbl Augenheilkd* 1997; 211(2): 94.
14. Krumeich JH, Schoner P, Lubatschowski H, Gerten G and Kermani O. Excimer laser treatment in deep lamellar keratoplasty 100 micrometer over Descemet's membrane. *Ophthalmologe* 2002; 99(12): 946.
15. Krumeich JH, Daniel J and Winter M. Depth of lamellar keratoplasty with the guided trephine system for transplantation of full-thickness donor sections. *Ophthalmologe* 1998; 95(11): 748.
16. Shimazaki J, Shimmura S, Ishioka M and Tsubota K. Randomized clinical trial of deep lamellar keratoplasty vs penetrating keratoplasty. *Am J Ophthalmol* 2002; 134(2): 159.
17. McDonald MB. Onlay lamellar keratoplasty. In: Kaufman HE, Barron BA and McDonald MB, *The Cornea*. Butterworth-Heinemann, Boston, 1998; 769.
18. Melles GR, Lander F, Beekhuis WH, Remeijer L and Binder PS. Posterior lamellar keratoplasty for a case of pseudophakic bullous keratopathy. *Am J Ophthalmol* 1999; 127(3): 340.
19. Melles GR, Lander F and Nieuwendaal C. Sutureless, posterior lamellar keratoplasty: a case report of a modified technique. *Cornea* 2002; 21(3): 325.
20. Barraquer JI. Full-thickness grafts. In: Rycroft BW, *Corneal Grafts*. Butterworth & Co, London, 1955; 86.
21. Barron BA. Penetrating keratoplasty. In: Kaufman HE, Barron BA and McDonald MB, *The Cornea*. Butterworth-Heinemann, Boston, 1998; 805.
22. Busin M. New suturing technique for stable post-PK corneal shape. *ESCRS Eurotimes* 2002; 7: 31.
23. Martin TP, Reed JW, Legault C *et al.* Cataract formation and cataract extraction after penetrating keratoplasty. *Ophthalmology* 1994; 101: 113.
24. Pineros OE, Cohen EJ, Rapuano CJ and Laibson PR. Triple vs nonsimultaneous procedures in Fuchs' dystrophy and cataract. *Arch Ophthalmol* 1996; 114: 525.
25. Malbran ES, Malbran E, Buonsanti J and Androgue E. Closed-system phacoemulsification and posterior chamber implant combined with penetrating keratoplasty. *Ophthalmic Surg* 1993; 24: 608.

26. Tsai RJ, Sun TT and Tseng SC. Comparison of limbal and conjunctival autograft transplantation in corneal surface reconstruction in rabbits. *Ophthalmology* 1990; 97(4): 446.
27. Nishiwaki-Dantas MC, Dantas PE and Reggi JR. Ipsilateral limbal translocation for treatment of partial limbal deficiency secondary to ocular alkali burn. *Br J Ophthalmol* 2001; 85(9): 1031.
28. Thoft RA. Keratoepithelioplasty. *Am J Ophthalmol* 1984; 97: 1.
29. Tsai RJ, Li L and Chen J. Reconstruction of damaged corneas by transplantation of autologous limbal epithelial cells. *Am J Ophthalmol* 2000; 130(4): 543.
30. Yao YF, Zhang B, Zhou P and Jiang JK. Autologous limbal grafting combined with deep lamellar keratoplasty in unilateral eye with severe chemical or thermal burn at late stage. *Ophthalmology* 2002; 109(11): 2011.
31. Holland EJ, Djalilian AR and Schwartz GS. Management of aniridic keratopathy with keratolimbal allograft: a limbal stem cell transplantation technique. *Ophthalmology* 2003; 110(1): 125.
32. Koizumi N, Inatomi T, Suzuki T, Sotozono C and Kinoshita S. Cultivated corneal epithelial stem cell transplantation in ocular surface disorders. *Ophthalmology* 2001; 108(9): 1569.
33. Pan Z, Zhang W, Wu Y and Sun B. Transplantation of corneal stem cells cultured on amniotic membrane for corneal burn: experimental and clinical study. *Chin Med J (Engl)* 2002; 115(5): 767.
34. Solomon A, Ellies P, Anderson DF, Touhami A, Grueterich M, Espana EM, Ti SE, Goto E, Feuer WJ and Tseng SC. Long-term outcome of keratolimbal allograft with or without penetrating keratoplasty for total limbal stem cell deficiency. *Ophthalmology* 2002; 109(6): 1159.
35. Hirst LW and Lee GA. Corneoscleral transplantation for end stage corneal disease. *Br J Ophthalmol* 1998; 82: 1276.
36. Krumeich JH and Daniel J. Perforating keratoplasty with an intracorneal ring. *Cornea* 1999; 18(3): 277.
37. Siganos D, Ferrara P, Chatzinikolas K, Bessis N and Papastergiou G. Ferrara intrastromal corneal rings for the correction of keratoconus. *J Cataract Refract Surg* 2002; 28(11): 1947.

3

The Clinical Problem

Introduction

By reputation corneal allografts in humans enjoy considerable success: survival rates for the first year are high [1] even in the absence of tissue typing. From early times it has been possible to obtain prolonged clarity of corneal allografts (see Chapter 1) and it is this which has spurred ophthalmic surgeons to improve the overall acceptance rate. However, recent audits of large series of cases have shown that the long term acceptance of corneal grafts in humans is less impressive [1] and may in fact be less than in other types of solid organ allograft such as the kidney [2]. It might be argued that this is because grafted corneas are not tissue matched while kidneys are, but tissue typing and matching is beneficial predominantly in preventing the direct alloresponse and has less effect on indirect alloresponses (see Chapter 5). Indirect alloresponses depend to some extent on the amount of donor "passenger" leukocytes present in the tissue; indirect presentation of processed alloantigen by host APCs is the basis of rejection of corneal allografts and of some cases of late, chronic rejection of other solid organ allografts, and is therefore likely to depend more on the amount of alloantigen present rather than on the frequency of allelic differences. Thus the relative similarity in late rejection rates for cornea and kidney (65% survival vs 71% survival at 5 years) [3] is not surprising given that the limitation on rejection depends on host processing of alloantigen and not on the level of "naturally" available alloreactive T cells as occurs with direct alloresponses.

The major clinical barrier to acceptance of an allograft therefore, for both unmatched corneal allografts and matched noncorneal allografts, is late rejection, assuming that technical problems associated with the surgery can be avoided and that factors associated either with ongoing innate immunity (e.g. inflammation in eyes with alkali burns, or herpes virus activity in the host) or with accelerated adaptive immunity (e.g. in presensitized hosts requiring second or third grafts) are absent.

Indications for Corneal Graft

The indications for corneal allograft depend not only on the presence of an opaque cornea but on many other factors which might appear initially to be of insufficient importance, such as the patient's ability to comply with good postoperative care, the general health and age of the patient, the cause of the corneal opacity, and the state of health of the eye and the fellow eye. Grafts may be performed for different fundamental reasons, e.g. for visual rehabilitation, to save the eye at risk of perforation of the cornea (the tectonic graft) or to relieve pain, e.g. in the case of recurrent corneal epithelial breakdown in bullous keratopathy (see Chapter 2).

The Eye Bank Association of America has defined several disease categories as indications for penetrating keratoplasty (Table 1).

Visual rehabilitation

Restoration of vision through replacement of an opaque cornea with a clear one is the major indication for corneal allografting. There are many causes and degrees of severity of corneal opacity and different surgeons have varying thresholds for recommending corneal grafting as therapy. This is frequently a consideration in cases of keratoconus where visual rehabilitation using a contact lens may be acceptable and well tolerated by some patients but not by others with the same degree of visual disability. In general a level of vision which significantly affects the individual quality of life of the patient and which cannot be corrected and/or tolerated with refraction or contact lens is taken as the main optical indication for corneal grafting. Consideration may also be taken of the basic refractive power of the eye

Table 1. Clinical indications for penetrating keratoplasty.

Bullous Keratopathy
Pseudophakic
Aphakic
Stromal Corneal Dystrophies
Primary Corneal Endotheliopathies
Corneal Ectasia/Thinning
Infectious Keratitis
Microbial: bacterial, fungal, chlamydial, parasitic
Viral: herpetic
Luetic: interstitial
Noninfectious Keratitis
Exposure
Autoimmune
Corneal Degenerations
Trauma
Chemical
Mechanical
Regraft
Postrejection
Postfailure
Miscellaneous
E.g. silicone keratopathy

when preparing the donor cornea, e.g. if the eye is aphakic or highly myopic and in these circumstances, "steep" or "flat" donor corneas respectively may be placed. However, it is more common to correct such problems with intraocular lenses of appropriate power. Lesser degrees of potential refractive problems postgraft can be corrected by selective removal of interrupted sutures in certain meridians as predicted by keratometry [4].

Pseudophakic bullous keratopathy has become a common indication for penetrating keratoplasty (PK) in the United States, mainly due to the early use of anterior chamber IOLs [5] while infectious causes of corneal scarring remain a major indication worldwide. Regraft also is an increasing indication in North America although the success rate diminishes with repeated regrafts [6, 7]. Keratoconus is the main noninfectious indication for corneal grafting outside the USA in both developed and less developed countries [8–10]. Cicatrizing corneal disease associated with ocular surface problems has a poor prognosis [11].

Preserving ocular integrity

Much less frequently it may be necessary to attempt to save an eye with loss of corneal tissue either from surgical or nonaccidental injury, or from inflammatory disease (corneal melt, e.g. in alkali burns or infective keratitis) by placing a graft. Spontaneous perforation of the cornea can occur for instance in alkali burns where there is ongoing inflammation, in eyes of patients with severe rheumatoid vasculitis and associated "melts" of the cornea and in patients with bacterial infective ulcers which penetrate

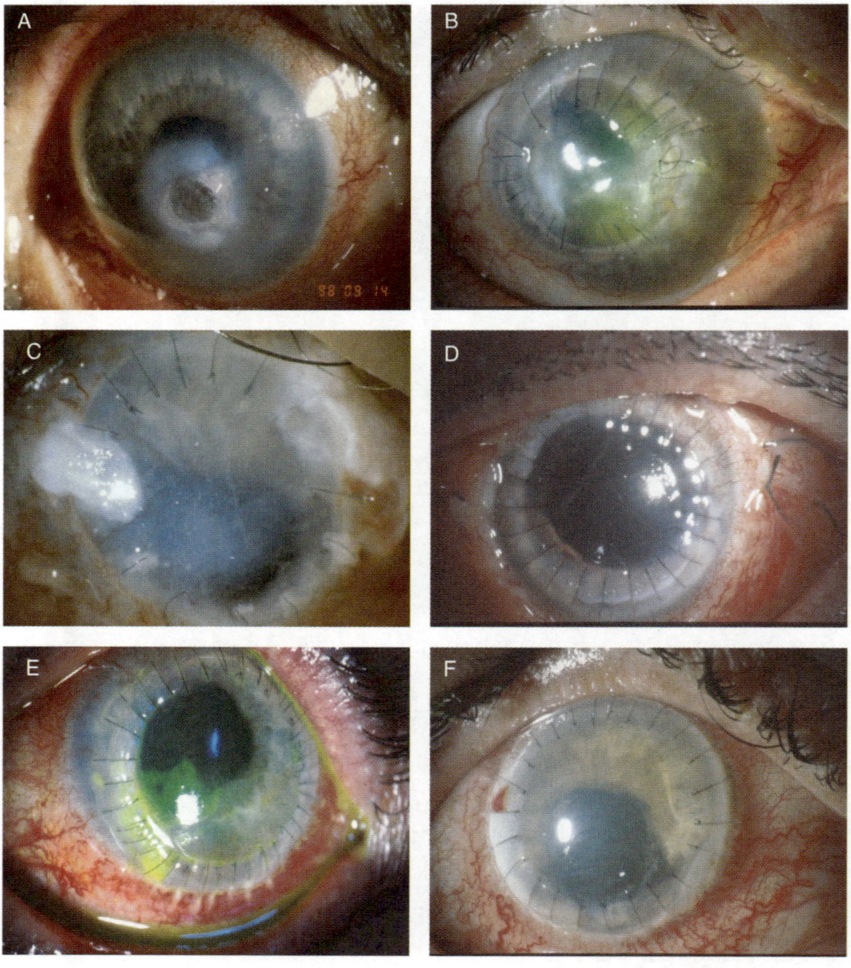

Figure 3.1 "Hot" eyes requiring treatment with tectonic sclerocorneal grafts. (**A**) A large descemetocele, which did not respond to treatment with polymethacrylate glue. (**B, C**) Corneal melts in patients with rheumatoid arthritis and alkali burn. (**D, E, F**) Examples of large corneal and sclerocorneal grafts. (*Courtesy M. Filipec.*)

deeply through the stroma and cause endophthalmitis (Figure 3.1). Grafts of this type are described as tectonic and may be large eccentric to cover a particular defect or even be combined with a part of the sclera (a sclero-corneal graft) if the corneal perforation involves the limbus. Full thickness, lamellar and "mushroom" grafts (mixed lamellar and full thickness grafts) have been used with success [12] and special techniques using a microkeratome and an artifical anterior chamber system have improved overall outcomes in some series [13] (Figure 3.2). In general the cure rate for bacterial

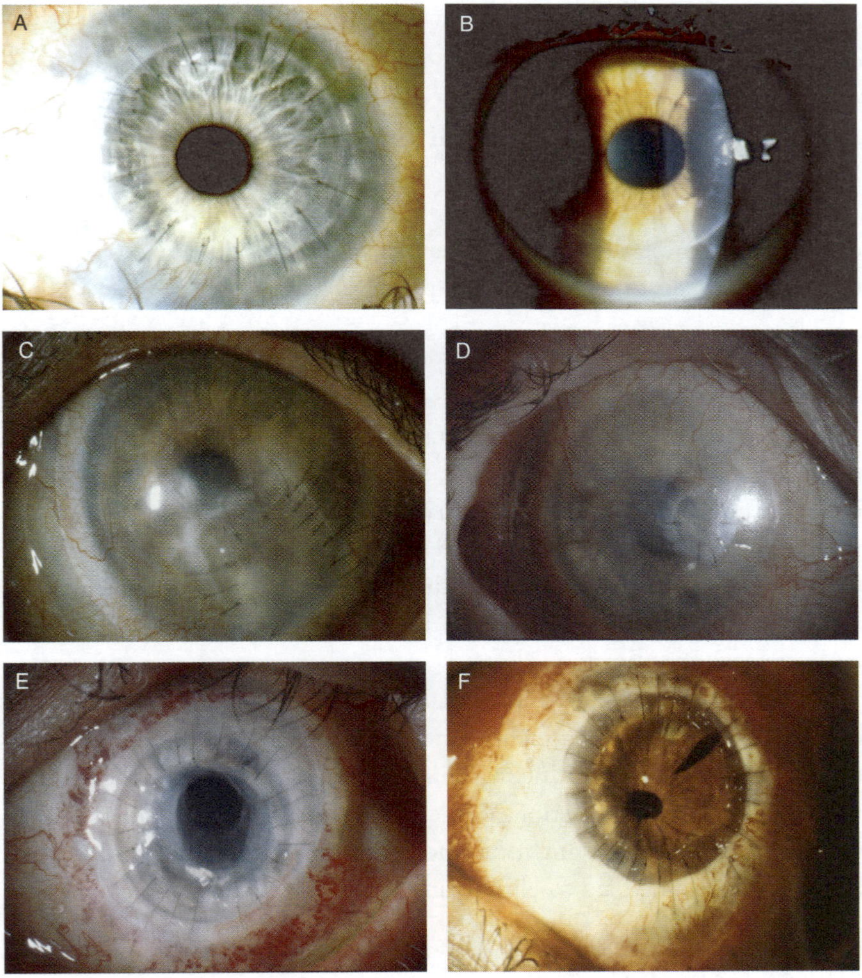

Figure 3.2 Types of corneal transplantation. (**A**) Full-thickness corneal transplantation with sutures *in situ*. (**B**) Full-thickness corneal transplantation after suture removal. (**C**) Lamellar keratoplasty. (**D**) Small—"patch" keratoplasty. (**E, F**) Full-thickness corneal transplantation with sutures *in situ* in association with limbal allograft. (*Courtesy M. Filipec.*)

infections is good but for parasitic acanthamoeba there is a tendency for recurrence [14].

Indications for combined procedures

Combined procedures involving lens extraction, anterior vitrectomy and insertion of an intraocular lens (see Chapter 2) are also performed in a significant proportion of cases when there is multiple ocular pathology. Such cases might include patients with extensive ocular surface disorders, alkali burns or other trauma although the prognosis for a good visual outcome is significantly reduced [11].

Contraindications for Corneal Graft

While certain patients may appear at first examination to be good candidates for corneal allografting, other considerations may finally persuade the surgeon against undertaking the procedure.

Ocular contraindications

As indicated above, there are certain obvious ocular conditions which militate against a successful outcome; for instance, repeated grafting in cases of graft failure or rejection ("high risk" grafts) have a reduced prognosis with each surgery, even if combined with favourable tissue matching (see Chapter 5). In addition, patients with severe ocular surface problems have a poor prognosis as do certain types of infectious keratitis such as postherpetic corneal opacification.

However, even relatively minor conditions may have a deleterious effect on outcomes. Conditions such as meibomitis, intercurrent conjunctivitis, unsuspected allergic eye disease, minor trauma and loosening of sutures may all initiate graft rejection. While not necessarily contraindications to grafting, they are important confounders in the preoperative work up and attention should be paid to eliminating these risk factors.

Nonocular contraindications

The after care of corneal graft requires a high level of awareness on the part of the surgeon and the patient, not only in compliance with topical and systemic treatment if required, but also in detecting the earliest symptoms and signs of graft rejection (see below). In addition, the home environment should be such that there is not undue exposure to the risk of infection and that appropriate hygienic practices are in place. This requires training and counselling of the patient and others who might be involved in the after care particularly with children and patients with learning disabilities. In the older patients there is greater likelihood of concomitant systemic disease such as rheumatological problems which may prevent good self care for instance in the use of topical medication. Due consideration therefore of these many associated factors may lead to a decision not the undertake PK in a particular patient.

Preoperative Work-up

An overall assessment of the patient's systemic and ocular health is essential in the preoperative evaluation for corneal graft. Detailed information is available in many texts and is briefly summarized here.

The following information should be obtained:

- Medical history, including cause of ocular condition
- Drug history
- Family history
- Ocular examination (vision, biomicroscopy of ocular surface and anterior segment, lens, presence of IOL, lens capsule, intraocular pressure, fundus exam if possible)
- Ocular imaging (e.g. ultrasound to evaluate the posterior segment)
- Electrophysiology, if considered necessary to determine defective retinal/optic nerve function but may not be very informative

In addition, it may be necessary to perform a range of general blood and radiology tests to determine whether there is any underlying cause to the corneal disease and whether the patient is suitable for systemic immunosuppression should this be required, e.g. in regraft patients (see Chapter 11).

Complications of Corneal Graft Surgery Affecting Graft Survival

In the immediate postgraft period, complications may arise which, while themselves not manifestations of rejection, have a bearing on the outcome of the graft success [15]. These include technical problems relating to the graft such as wound leaks or dehiscence; in addition, surface problems in the host may compromise the epithelium and lead to persistent epithelial defects or to a filamentary keratitis, which probably represents rolled epithelial sheets failing to adhere to the donor surface as occurs in dry eye disease. Control of postoperative inflammation is critical to the eventual survival of the graft and is usually well managed with topical corticosteroids. As with experimental corneal grafts, there is a tendency to fibrin formation in the anterior chamber, sometimes of sufficient severity to require treatment with tPA. Fibrin deposition is the main inducer of anterior synechiae, which are also a major negative factor for graft survival, clinically and experimentally [16]. Late spontaneous dehiscence may occur in about 7% of cases after removal of a continuous suture [17].

Other complications which may indirectly affect graft outcome are raised intraocular pressure sometimes due to pupillary block, and more

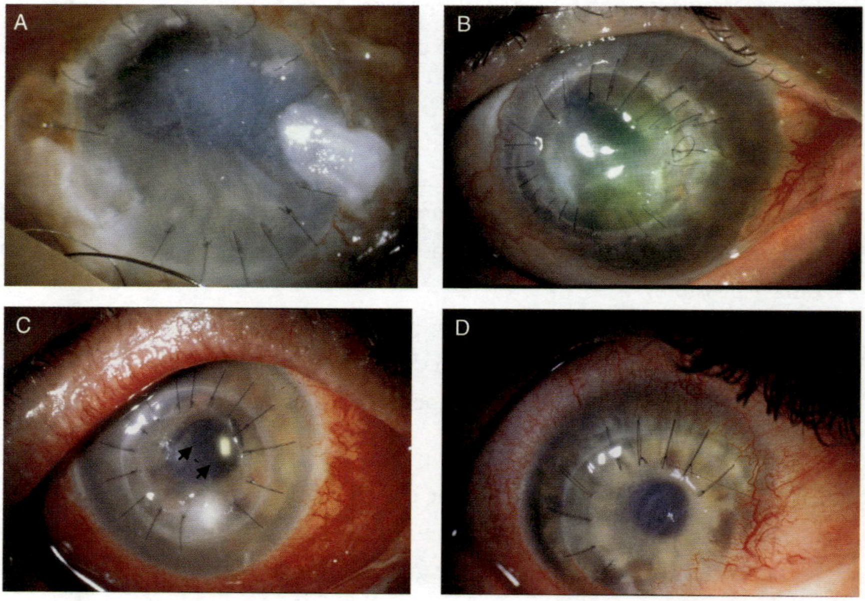

Figure 3.3 Suture-related complications. (**A**) Loose corneal sutures in a case of advanced corneal tissue melting associated with alkali burn. (**B**) Loose corneal sutures inducing corneal neovascularization. (**C**) Suture-associated microabscess; arrows delineate advancing edge of endothelial rejection line. (**D**) Suture-induced neovascularization on the donor graft and recipient cornea persisting after suture removal. Note suture-related microabscesses at 7–8 o'clock meridian. (*Courtesy M. Filipec.*)

severe complications like anterior chamber haemorrhage (hyphaema), choroidal haemorrhage and detachment, and fixed dilated pupil.

Suture complications are common including loose sutures sometimes leading to wound leak, suture exposure, suture-associated infection (microabscesses), and foreign body reactions ("immune infiltrates") (Figure 3.3). Frank infection of the graft may occur, including endophthalmitis, usually within 24–48 h of surgery (see Chapter 12) and is heralded by pain, ciliary injection (pericorneal redness), oedema and opacity of the graft and a mucopurulent discharge.

Finally, primary graft failure may occur. This is manifested by graft opacification from day 1 postoperatively which does not improve with time. It is more likely to occur when the donor corneal endothelium has been compromised either through poor preservation or surgical trauma but may also occur in donor grafts which harbour infective material (see Chapter 12).

Although not exactly a complication, recurrence of stromal dystrophy, especially granular and lattice dystrophies some years after grafting, is not infrequent and requires to be considered in any plans for PK [18].

Symptoms and Signs of Corneal Allograft Rejection in Humans

Irreversible corneal graft rejection in humans is usually preceded by one of more "rejection episodes". Unlike in the study of experimental graft rejection where immunosuppressants are not routinely used unless they are part of a specific study, it is standard practice in human corneal grafts to administer topical steroids in the immediate postoperative phase and to continue this therapy for as long as is necessary to keep the eye "quiet". In addition, since corneal vascularization is known to be associated with graft rejection, evidence of new vessels which usually occurs around sutures is normally rapidly dealt with by topical steroid application; any intervention which is likely to stimulate a further inflammatory response such as removal of sutures is also "covered" by use of topical steroids. Therefore the natural course of graft rejection in humans is modified by use of local immunosuppressant steroids and may be delayed, prevented or treated by such management.

In spite of this, irreversible graft rejection occurs and usually in eyes which have been considered "quiet", are "off" topical steroid therapy and in which the early symptoms and signs of rejection have been ignored either by the patient or by the physician.

Rejection episodes

Rejection episodes are short periods of time when part or all of the donor cornea is under immunological attack which come to an end after appropriate treatment and are followed by full recovery of corneal clarity and function.

Patients are often the first to recognize problems in a graft by experience of symptoms of photophobia, redness, slightly decreased vision and discomfort/ache/throbbing which persists for some time e.g. hours or days [19]. These symptoms need not necessarily indicate rejection of the graft.

Signs of a rejection episode are often subtle. The appearance of ciliary flush may precede infiltration of cells in the anterior chamber. Aqueous humour flare (turbidity) is a late sign of rejection (Figure 3.4A, B).

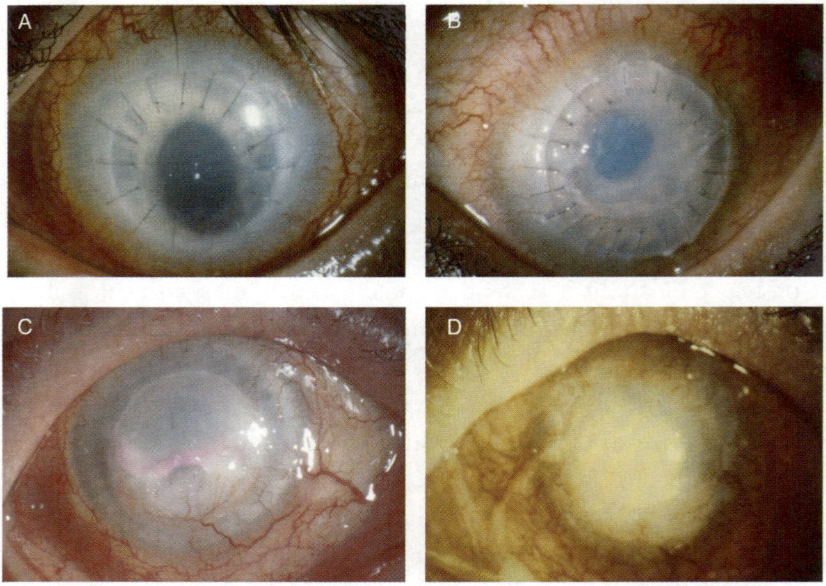

Figure 3.4 Acute rejection episode and chronic rejection-graft failure. (**A, B**) Acute corneal graft rejection associated with ciliary injection, keratic precipitates on donor endothelium and slightly oedematous corneal graft. (**C**) Opaque, failed corneal graft with 180° extent of neovascularization representing "high risk" recipient for a subsequent corneal grafting; note meibomitis on upper eyelid. (**D**) Dense corneal leucoma after failed corneal transplantation with the impression of IOL beneath the failed graft. (*Courtesy M. Filipec.*)

Cells in the aqueous are characteristically very small and discrete and are easily missed. Keratic precipitates represent an ongoing inflammation which has been of sufficient duration (hours to days) to allow cells to adhere to the endothelium and is a definitive sign of rejection.

Irreversible graft rejection

More aggressive signs of inflammation are a poor prognostic sign for graft survival. Infiltrates of cells may occur in the epithelium, the stroma or on the endothelium. Early punctate subepithelial infiltrates may occur in isolation and may be reversible but are more usually associated with irreversible changes. Epithelial rejection is characterized by a rejection line and represents replacement of the donor epithelium by host cells; this is usually not a sign of irreversible rejection. However, similar endothelial rejection lines (termed Khodadoust lines; see Chapter 8) indicate irreversible rejection of the graft. Such lines usually develop close to an area of vascularization and progress inexorably across the cornea (Figure 3.3C). If vascularization is circumferential, the line develops as a circle which becomes progressively smaller and disappears in the centre of the cornea leaving an opaque or at best a translucent donor graft. Histological studies in rabbits have shown that these lines are composed of advancing lymphocytes and macrophages which progress over and destroy healthy endothelium leaving in their wake a denuded Descemet's membrane sparsely covered by residual fibroblast-like cells and inflammatory cells (see Chapter 8).

Evidence of endothelial rejection lines are not essential for a diagnosis of irreversible rejection. Scattered keratic precipitates are probably more common and also more difficult to evaluate in terms of the prognosis for the graft. In other circumstances, the process may be well advanced before recognition of rejection and the line has passed. Deep stromal vascularization is a sign to be considered, especially focal vessels.

Historically, late opacification of a graft after a period of clarity was described as graft failure, but was later shown to be due to sensitization of the donor cornea to the host and was then considered to be graft rejection (for review see Ref. 20) (Figure 3.4C, D). Primary graft failure now is a term usually applied to opacification of the graft from the time of surgery (see above); clinically it is often difficult to differentiate late graft failure from irreversible graft rejection and similar conundrums apply to other solid organ grafts [3]. Occasionally, recurrence of herpetic disease in a donor cornea may mimic graft rejection and can particularly be induced by the excessive use of topical steroids to control inflammation. In addition, the possibility of low grade infection of the graft by opportunistic organisms must be considered. Pathophysiologically, a failed graft has a nonfunctioning endothelium as has an irreversibly rejected one, so the perceived difference may be a semantic one.

Factors Affecting Clinical Rejection

Probably the most important factor in predicting outcome of PK is the condition of the recipient cornea. Clearly, a tectonic graft placed into an inflamed eye is not expected to function visually, is likely to become opaque and is thus technically "rejected", but has served the purpose for which it was intended, i.e. to preserve the integrity of the globe.

In contrast, PK performed for visual purposes is considered rejected or "failed" (see above), if it loses transparency. Several factors contribute to an increasing risk of rejection and recipients with a poor prognosis are considered "high risk". Factors affecting this are many. For instance different types of graft develop opacity at different rates (e.g. full thickness grafts are more at risk then lamellar because the endothelium is the main determinant of corneal transparency). In addition, larger grafts are more likely to reject than small grafts partly because they are closer to the limbus and thus more likely to induce neovascularization. There are also the theoretical possibilities that they contain greater numbers of passenger leukocytes (dendritic cells) and are thus likely to induce a direct as well as an indirect alloresponse (see Chapter 6).

Certain factors, therefore, can predict the likelihood of the potential allograft reaction [21]. These include:

(a) The degree of prevascularization of the recipient bed;
(b) The size of the donor corneal button;
(c) The position of the donor corneal button in the recipient bed;
(d) Preservation methods for the donor cornea;
(e) The choice of immunosuppression;
(f) The immune status of the recipient's cornea;
(g) Immunohistocompatibilities between donor and recipient;
(h) The age of the recipient—younger recipients are less successful than older recipients;
(i) Previous corneal failure due to rejection.

The last point is particularly important, because it has been shown that patients who have had previous graft failure from rejection have a greater than 50% chance of subsequent failure and these reactions occur more rapidly and with a more fulminant course. Failure is directly correlated with the severity of corneal vascularization [22].

The surgical technique (see Chapter 2) has an important bearing on the outcome of graft surgery. This reflects the induction of the innate immune response: it is increasingly recognized that the severity of the innate immune response in part determines the strength of the adaptive immune response. Results of the large series of prospective clinical studies have shown that the skill and experience of the surgeon have an influence on the outcome. For instance, it is known that wound leaks in the early postoperative period are a poor prognosticator for graft survival; that poor suturing technique leading to loosening of the sutures and focal vascularization are associated with rejection; and that excessive handling of the donor graft reduces its likelihood of survival.

Finally, the question of tissue typing (HLA and ABO blood group matching) has a bearing on outcome although not as clearly as with vascularized organ grafts (see Chapter 5).

Conclusion

In summary, the major challenge faced by the corneal graft surgeon is to achieve a good visual outcome. Graft rejection is the main obstacle preventing this result and much remains to be learned concerning the mechanism of allorecognition of corneal grafts (see Chapter 6). With further knowledge, newer approaches to prevention of rejection can be developed. This applies particularly to the problem of the "high risk" graft.

In addition, the separate problem of graft failure, although not so frequent, should be recognized. In renal transplant studies it is now recognized that factors relating to the donor organ affect its function as a graft, as shown in "pairing" studies of kidney function after grafting [23]. Similar studies in corneal graft might provide useful information relating to donor-related factors affecting eventual visual outcome.

Future directions for clinical studies therefore should be aimed at identifying and minimizing the full range of risk factors. Since the biggest challenge relates to the "high risk" graft, experimental models investigating the immune mechanisms in high risk grafts should be developed. Finally, research in xenografting should also be encouraged since the problem of donor supply is only likely to become greater in the future.

References

1. Williams KA *et al.* How successful is corneal transplantation? A report from the Australian Corneal Graft Register. *Eye* 1995; 9(Pt 2): 219.
2. Williams KA *et al.* Long-term outcome in corneal allotransplantation: The Australian Corneal Graft Registry. *Transplant Proc* 1997; 29(1–2): 983.
3. Gourishankar S and Halloran PF. Late deterioration of organ transplants: a problem in injury and homeostasis. *Curr Opin Immunol* 2002; 14(5): 576.
4. Dursun D, Forster RK and Feuer WJ. Suturing technique for control of postkeratoplasty astigmatism and myopia. *Trans Am Ophthalmol Soc* 2002; 100: 51; discussion 57.
5. Cosar CB *et al.* Indications for penetrating keratoplasty and associated procedures, 1996–2000; *Cornea* 2002; 21(2): 148.
6. Maeno A *et al.* Three decades of corneal transplantation: indications and patient characteristics. *Cornea* 2000; 19(1): 7.
7. Patel NP *et al.* Indications for and outcomes of repeat penetrating keratoplasty, 1989–1995. *Ophthalmology* 2000; 107(4): 719.
8. Legeais JM *et al.* Nineteen years of penetrating keratoplasty in the Hotel-Dieu Hospital in Paris. *Cornea* 2001; 20(6): 603.
9. Edwards M *et al.* Indications for corneal transplantation in New Zealand: 1991–1999. *Cornea* 2002; 21(2): 152.
10. Mkanganwi N, Nondo SI and Guramatunhu S. Indications for corneal grafting in Zimbabwe. *Cent Afr J Med* 2000; 46(11): 300.
11. Tugal-Tutkun I, Akova YA and Foster CS. Penetrating keratoplasty in cicatrizing conjunctival diseases. *Ophthalmology* 1995; 102(4): 576.
12. Vanathi M *et al.* Tectonic grafts for corneal thinning and perforations. *Cornea* 2002; 21(8): 792.
13. Wiley LA, Joseph MA, and Springs, CL. Tectonic lamellar keratoplasty utilizing a microkeratome and an artificial anterior chamber system. *Cornea* 2002; 21(7): 661.
14. Sony P *et al.* Therapeutic keratoplasty for infectious keratitis: a review of the literature. *Clao J* 2002; 28(3): 111.
15. Chang SD *et al.* Factors influencing graft clarity. *Cornea* 1996; 15(6): 577.
16. Yamagami S. and Tsuru T. Increase in orthotopic murine corneal transplantation rejection rate with anterior synechiae. *Invest Ophthalmol Vis Sci* 1999; 40(10): 2422.
17. Abou-Jaoude ES *et al.* Spontaneous wound dehiscence after removal of single continuous penetrating keratoplasty suture. *Ophthalmology* 2002; 109(7): 1291; discussion 1297.
18. Marcon AS *et al.* Recurrence of corneal stromal dystrophies after penetrating keratoplasty. *Cornea* 2003; 22(1): 19.
19. Kamp MT *et al.* Patient-reported symptoms associated with graft reactions in high-risk patients in the collaborative corneal transplantation studies: Collaborative Corneal Transplantation Studies Research Group. *Cornea* 1995; 14(1): 43.

20. Maumenee AE. The Pocklington lecture, 1976: Recent advances in corneal transplantation. *Trans Ophthalmol Soc UK* 1976; 46(4): 462.
21. Katami M Corneal transplantation—immunologically privileged status. *Eye* 1991; 5 (Pt 5): 528.
22. Khodadoust AA and Silverstein AM. Studies on the nature of the privilege enjoyed by corneal allografts. *Invest Ophthalmol* 1972; 11(3): 137.
23. Gourishankar S *et al.* Donor tissue characteristics influence cadaver kidney transplant function and graft survival but not rejection. *J Am Soc Nephrol* 2003; 14(2): 493.

4

Eye Banking

Introduction

During the last 50 years advances in corneal tissue harvesting, preservation and distribution under the supervision of a worldwide network of eye banks allowed an increase in the numbers of surgeons performing full-thickness penetrating keratoplasties and also helped to prolong survival of such treated corneal grafts.

History

The first successful full-thickness penetrating keratoplasty in a human was performed in 1905 by Eduard Konrad Zirm (see Chapter 1) [1]. At that time the unaffected, fresh cornea from the otherwise damaged eye of an 11-year-old boy was retrieved and used to provide tissue for bilateral grafts for a patient whose eyes had been damaged by lime burns. One of the grafts remained clear for several years.

In the early 1930s, the first use of cadaver corneas was reported by Filatov [2]. He obtained whole eyes shortly after death, rinsed the globes in brilliant green solution, stored them at 4°C in a moist chamber and transplanted them within 56 hours. Later, in 1944, the first eye bank in the United States—the Eye Bank for Sight Restoration—was established by R. Townley Paton [3]. Since that time a series of corneal banks have been founded around the world.

As a result, a variety of methods for preservation of cadaver corneas were tested. Techniques such as tissue drying, formalin fixation, freezing, freeze-drying and liquid paraffin storage were unsuccessful and use of such treated corneas led to the failure of the corneal grafts [3, 4].

In the early 1950s, Stocker was the first scientist who recognized the crucial role of corneal endothelium for maintaining clarity of the cornea [5]. Since that time, research has been directed towards techniques which can protect and prolong the viability of corneal endothelial cells.

Cryopreservation as a method for achieving long-term preservation, was investigated extensively during the 1950s. The first successful transplantation in a human with a cryopreserved cornea was published by Eastcott *et al.* They pretreated corneas with glycerol and consequently froze them in a mixture of alcohol and carbon dioxide. Despite this there was considerable tissue damage due to the process of freezing and it was not for another 10 years that the use of dimethyl sulfoxide as an agent for cryopreservation was introduced. A technique reported by Capella *et al.* [6] used increasing concentrations of dimethyl sulfoxide followed by freezing of the tissue which allowed storage of the tissue for up to one year. Unfortunately the thawing procedure was technically demanding, due to the fact that dimethyl sulfoxide is toxic for endothelial cells at temperatures approaching 37°C. As a result, endothelial cell viability was less than optimal. Although this technique was used in some cornea banks, later it was replaced by simpler methods (i.e. intermediate and long-term preservative media; see below).

The modern approach to eye-banking started in 1974 when McCarey–Kaufman (M–K) medium was developed [7]. This solution comprised tissue culture medium, dextran, antibiotics and buffer which allowed corneas to be stored up to four days at 4°C. A few years later an organ-culture technique was introduced. This technique uses long-term preservative media, which allows storage of the corneas in 37°C for more than 30 days at 4°C. The major additional component of preservative medium was chondroitin sulphate [8]. Although the originally proposed medium containing chondroitin sulphate is no longer available, the derivatives of this formula (Optisol and Dextol) are used by cornea banks around the world.

Criteria for Cornea Donation

In the United States, the Eye Bank Association of America has set strict standards for corneal donation. The document, which is renewed annually, is approved by the Eye Banking Committee of the American Academy of Ophthalmology. In Europe a new Europe-wide law to regulate harvesting, testing and transplant of the tissue, including the eye was proposed recently [9] and it is recommended that all EU countries should introduce comprehensive standards to ensure the safety of tissue donations, the quality of tissue banks and traceability of tissue.

Donation of corneal tissue is excluded when the cause of death is unknown or in circumstances that could place the tissue recipient at risk from disease or infection. Such circumstances include situations where the donor:

(1) is known to have ingested or was exposed to a toxic substance that may be transmitted in a sufficient dose to the tissue recipients.
(2) has died from retinoblastoma, malignant melanoma of the anterior segment of the eye, haematological neoplasm and malignant tumor, which could affect the anterior segment of the eye.
(3) had active ocular or intraocular inflammation, congenital or acquired conditions, which could preclude a successful outcome of penetrating keratoplasty and pterygia, which involve central cornea.
(4) had a history of refractive surgery or laser photoablative surgery. If there was previous surgery to the anterior segment of the eye (cataract and antiglaucoma surgery), the cornea needs to be screened by specular microscopy and endothelial viability needs to meet standards of the eye bank.
(5) may have contracted a prion-induced disease, including confirmed and suspected cases of Creutzfeldt–Jakob Disease (CJD), and nonvariant CJD, progressive multifocal leukoencephalopathy, the human form of bovine spongiform encephalopathy, or so-called "mad cow" disease.
(6) had a history of rapid progressive dementia or degenerative neurological disease of unknown origin.
(7) had congenital rubella, rabies or active viral encephalitis.
(8) died of Reyes syndrome.
(9) had received pituitary gland-derived human growth hormones or dura matter.
(10) died of uncontrolled infection.

(11) had a history, clinical evidence, or confirmed positive laboratory test of HIV infection, acute or chronic hepatitis B or hepatitis C infection.
(12) had a history of chronic haemodialysis.

Under the proposed Europe-wide law, the Human Tissue Directive states that any doctor who harvests tissue will be required to create a dossier to accompany the tissue [9]. The dossier will contain:

(1) donor identification.
(2) the consent form from relatives of the deceased.
(3) clinical data relating to the donor.
(4) date and time of starting and ending the procurement of tissue.
(5) laboratory tests results.
(6) autopsy results, if any.

The clinical records of the donor must be kept for at least 30 years.

EU countries will be required to ensure that "all tissues and cells procured, processed, stored and distributed on their territory can be traced from the donor to recipient and vice versa". As part of the traceability program, each donation and its products will receive a unique identification code, which will be written on any packaging containing the tissue. The tissue banks will maintain tissue registers to which it will enter information about any tissue it has processed. The register will record:

(1) details of the consent to the donation.
(2) donor identification and characteristics: type of donor, age, sex, cause of death and presence of risk factors.
(3) review of clinical data against donor selection criteria.
(4) results of physical examination, laboratory tests and other tests (autopsy report where one was conducted).
(5) date and time of the death.
(6) date and time of the procurement and health care establishment where the procurement was carried out.
(7) conditions under which the cadaver was kept: refrigerated (or not), time of onset of refrigeration and time of transfer to procurement site.
(8) place of procurement, procurement team and person in charge of procurement.
(9) degree of asepsis.
(10) details of the preservation solutions used during procurement, including composition, lot, date of expiry, temperature, amount, concentration and preparation method.

(11) grafts obtained and relevant characteristics.
(12) relevant incidents that have occurred before, during and after procurement.
(13) destination of the tissue procured.
(14) method of preservation until arrival of tissues at the bank.

There are some special considerations concerning cornea donations. Although donors after refractive surgery or laser photoablative surgery usually have healthy endothelium, the shape and thickness of the cornea has been changed. The use of such treated corneas can result in high hyperopia in the recipient and therefore donor corneas treated with these forms of ocular surgery in the past are contraindicated for donation.

The upper and the lower age limit are not arbitrarily defined. Several studies showed a decrease in endothelial cell density, changes in size and shape of the endothelial cells and alteration of endothelial cell function with age. However, clinical studies have found no correlation between donor age and clarity of the transplanted cornea. Therefore most clinical directors of eye banks have established an upper age limit between 60 and 75 years. However, it is preferable that the donor is not considerably older than the recipient, especially in the case of the recipient-child.

The infant cornea is unusually steep with an average curvature of approximately 50 diopters. Several studies have noted high myopia after transplantation of such corneas [10]. Although some authors suggest the use of infant corneas to correct refractive errors such as aphakia, a more common approach to aphakia is secondary implantation of an intraocular lens into the lens capsule, fixated into the iridociliary sulcus or placed into the anterior chamber of the eye (see Chapter 2). The infant cornea and the cornea from young individuals are also very malleable and have a tendency to fold over on themselves, which results in damage to the endothelium. For all these reasons the use of such donor corneas should be left only for emergency situations.

Agreement between eye banks on the maximal time for acceptable donor viability postmortem to enucleation is not universal. Criteria are generally set by medical directors of each eye bank, but in the main, it is recommended to enucleate the donor eye within six hours postmortem due to the fact that decomposition of uveal and other intraocular tissues into the aqueous humour generates a highly toxic environment for corneal endothelial cells. The local changes in pH, decrease in glucose and oxygen concentrations, increase in potassium and lactate concentrations and released lysosomal proteases from dead and dying cells all have adverse effects on quality and viability of endothelial cells.

Procurement and Examination of Donor Corneas

Following the correct procedure for tissue procurement is the first and most important step towards obtaining high quality donor corneal tissue. There are in essence two techniques for cornea procurement: (a) enucleation of the entire globe with later corneal trephination and dissection from an anterior route and (b) excision of donor cornea/sclera from the retained donor eye with later trephination and dissection of the corneal button usually from an endothelial route [11].

Enucleation starts with preparation of a sterile field: the conjunctival fornices are washed out with antibiotics and saline. A 360° limbal peritomy is made with disruption of all adhesions between the Tenon's fascia and sclera. The extraocular muscles are separated and detached from the eye. The optic nerve is severed with long, curved enucleation scissors and the intact globe is removed from the orbit. The enucleated eye is placed into a moist chamber and flooded with antibiotics solution.

The majority of eye banks use short-term or intermediate-term preservation medium, which requires removal of the cornea with a rim of sclera from the enucleated eye. For this reason some eye banks recommend to remove donor cornea and sclera *in situ* in the donor orbit (see above) [12]. This procedure is commenced with a full-thickness incision in the sclera 3 mm behind the limbus with a blade. Scissors are used to extend the incision up to 360°. Attention is paid to cut only the sclera and not underlying structures. The scleral edge is lifted and separated from attachments with iris and choroid. The anterior chamber is opened and cornea with a 3-mm-wide scleral rim is removed from the eye and placed into the preservative medium.

The enucleated eye should be examined with a slit lamp to detect any corneal abnormalities, such as the presence of neovascularization, which can render the cornea unsuitable for transplantation. The next step is specular microscopy, which can reveal abnormalities in the shape and size of endothelial cells and endothelial cell density. There are some limitations to the use of specular microscopy. For instance, if the corneal epithelium and stroma are swollen due to the presence of postmortem oedema, the view of the endothelium may be poor. To resolve such difficulties, confocal microscopy may be useful as a standard technique for checking the endothelium in the future.

Techniques for Assessing Endothelial Cell Viability

Techniques which assess endothelial cell viability, either directly or indirectly, achieve their function by evaluating changes in cell morphology and in specific metabolic processes.

Staining techniques employed include use of dyes such as trypan blue, alizarin red and nitroblue tetrazolium or other fluorescent dyes to differentiate viable and nonviable endothelial cells. Trypan blue is directly applied to the cornea for a couple of minutes and then rinsed off. The stain penetrates only nonviable cells, which absorb the dye through damaged plasma membranes and stains the nucleus [13]. The percentage of nonviable endothelial cells is counted under the light microscope. Trypan blue staining can be combined with alizarin red staining, which highlights the intracellular space of damaged cells. The major disadvantage of such staining is that the dye stains both damaged and dead cells, and gives a false impression of total cell death since some damaged cells have the potential to recover and re-establish viability. Severely damaged endothelial cells do not take up trypan blue staining.

Nitroblue tetrazolium is reduced by enzymes released from endothelial cells (dehydrogenases and diaphorases). Therefore positive staining with this dye occurs in areas of enzyme release around nonviable cells [14].

Acridine orange is a fluorescent dye, which can penetrate the plasma membrane of viable cells and stains double-stranded DNA [15]. In combination with ethidium bromide, the dyes penetrate only nonviable cells and allow easy differentiation between viable and nonviable endothelial cells. This staining has to be viewed under the fluorescent microscope. The advantage of these staining procedures is that they are technically not too demanding. The disadvantage is that differentiation between dead and damaged, but viable, cells which have the potential for recovery is difficult and thus at the time of monitoring a larger than true area of nonviability is observed. On this basis certain corneas which are useful may arbitrarily be rejected.

Tests of endothelial cell function can also be used to assess viability of a donor graft. A somewhat rudimentary test is the "temperature reversal technique", which uses the reversible thinning phenomenon of the cornea that is observed when the cornea is rewarmed after cooling [16]. In this case, the thickness of the cornea is measured by specular microscopy. This technique is a measure of the metabolic and physiological fluid pumping functions of the endothelial monolayer, which is a primary condition for corneal graft survival.

Morphological tests are also useful. The use of transmission electron microscopy can reveal changes in subcellular morphology. Changes such as intracellular vacuolization, mitochondrial swelling, damage of plasma and nuclear membrane structures, changes in nuclear matrix and chromatin, and disruption of intercellular adhesions and hemidesmosome attachments to Descemet's membrane can indicate signs of cellular damage [17]. The limitation of the use of this technique is the high cost of equipment and confusions with artifacts due to the high power and small visualization field.

Specular microscopy is the most commonly used morphological technique for monitoring effective corneal preservation [18]. Endothelial cell density, changes in size or shape of the cells and estimation of the number of sides per cells (corneal endothelial cells normally have a hexagonal appearance (Figure 4.1)) can be determined in enucleated eyes and also on dissected corneas. The major advantage of this technique is the opportunity

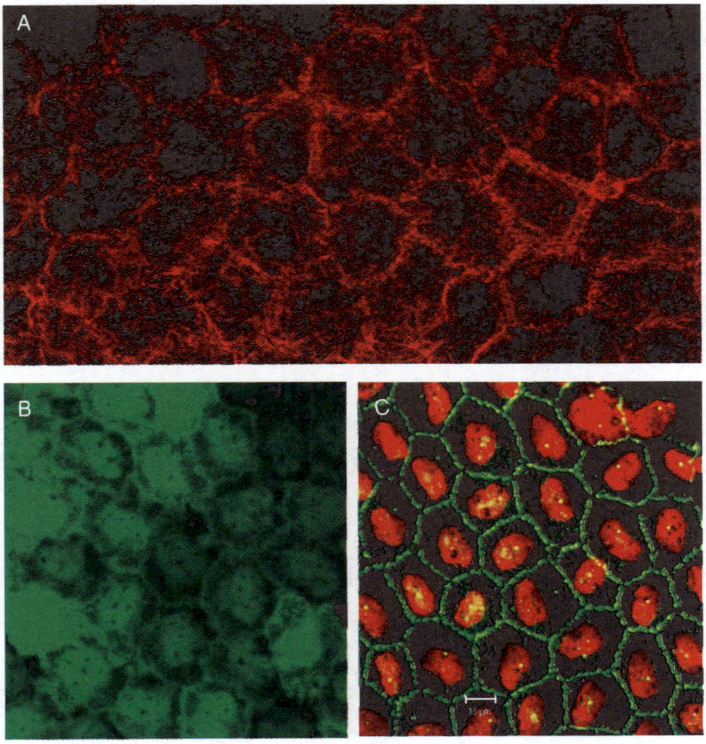

Figure 4.1 Corneal endothelial cell monolayer visualized by: (**A**) actin staining; (**B**) green fluorescent protein in the GFP-transgenic mouse; note the interlocking junctions; (**C**) dual staining of the intercellular adhesion protein, *zonula occludens* [ZO-1; green – FITC] and nuclei with propidium iodide (PI). (*Figure 4.1C courtesy H. Xu.*)

to compare endothelial cell density before corneal transplantation with *in situ* cell density after the surgery. The limitation of the technique is that it is technically difficult—a well-trained technician and appropriate equipment are required. The comparison of the corneas before and after the grafting procedure has to take into account loss of endothelial cells from the graft-recipient border due to the surgical manipulation. These cells are replaced by enlargement and spreading of donor endothelial cells from the center of the graft which results in changes in the specular microscopy appearance even in the absence of cell loss due to the corneal preservative. The optimum time to perform specular microscopy post corneal transplantation is two months after surgery when the cornea is still clear. There are difficulties in assessing the endothelial cell density in swollen, oedematous corneal grafts. In the future the confocal scanning ophthalmoscope can be used for scanning the endothelial layer through the oedematous corneal stroma since it is possible that endothelial cell density and cell morphology may be relatively intact in certain circumstances of corneal opacity (see Chapter 8).

The crystal-clear corneal graft is the ultimate goal of patient, surgeon and scientists involved in research on corneal preservation. Unfortunately clinical observation is not a sufficiently sensitive measure of the efficacy of corneal preservation techniques. Transplanted corneas with initial low numbers of viable endothelial cells have a greater tendency and possibility to fail in the long-term due to the further cell loss associated with age, immunological insults—rejection episodes, trauma, glaucoma or simple normal attrition. Therefore, the main aim is to provide corneal tissue with the highest possible numbers of viable endothelial cells.

Methods of Corneal Preservation

The major aims in methods for corneal preservation are (1) to maintain the highest possible numbers of viable donor endothelial cells, keratocytes and epithelial cells using the simplest preservative medium, and (2) to prevent microbial contamination of the donor tissue (see Chapter 12).

The oldest (and simplest) method of corneal storage is the moist chamber. The closed moist chamber is filled with a small amount of saline to moisten the air around the enucleated eye, and stored in 4°C. This technique is limited by a short preservation time and it is generally accepted that the maximum storage time should not exceed 48 hours. At that time the corneal endothelium is exposed to unfavourable postmortem conditions in the anterior chamber of the enucleated eye. Changes in electrolyte balance, low or depleted oxygen and glucose, and increased lactic acid and potassium are toxic for the endothelium and compromise its viability. Studies performed on human eyes, which were stored in the moist chamber, revealed 44% loss of viable endothelium after 48 hours in 4°C [19]. Storage in the moist chamber can also be potentially dangerous, if there is a risk that the temperature rises above 4°C, since there are then increased metabolic demands and due to the lack of nutrients and oxygen, the endothelium cannot survive.

Cryopreservation is a technique which offers indefinite preservation of corneal tissue [20]. Unfortunately, so far there is no fully developed technically simple method for cryopreservation, which is simultaneously effective in maintaining endothelial cell viability. The cryopreservation technique, which was clinically tested, is similar to the original technique published by Capella *et al.* and O'Neill *et al.* [6, 21, 22]. The cornea should be collected within eight hours postmortem and then placed into a very dilute solution of dimethyl sulfoxide with continually increasing concentrations. The final concentration of dimethyl sulfoxide is 7.5% and then tissue has to be deep frozen in liquid nitrogen at –80°C and stored at –196°C. Rather difficult is the thawing process, where the thawing temperature has to be carefully monitored due to the fact that dimethyl sulfoxide is toxic for endothelial cells at temperatures higher than 37°C. The major limitation of this technique is the low efficacy in preserving viable corneal endothelium [23, 24]. This loss has been attributed to increased concentrations of dimethyl sulfoxide, formation of ice crystals and changes in pH and osmolality [25]. Clinical study has reported that on average, corneas treated by cryopreservation required a longer time to clear than those stored in the moist chamber or M–K medium.

The use of short-term or intermediate-term preservative medium is another method for preserving corneal tissue. The first short-term medium for corneal storage was proposed in 1974 by McCarey and Kaufman and contained tissue culture medium TC-199, dextran, bicarbonate buffer and gentamicin [7]. The current formulation contains HEPES buffer instead of bicarbonate buffer and phenol red as pH indicator. This medium was designed for storage of donor corneas for up to four days in 4°C. The superiority of M–K medium to moist chamber storage, particularly after 48 hours, has been demonstrated in numerous studies using trypan blue, electron microscopy and specular microscopy. Clinical studies have also reported good success with corneas stored in M–K medium [26].

Intermediate-term storage medium contains chondroitin sulphate and can be used for storage of donor corneas up to 14 days at 4°C. The K-Sol, developed by Kaufman, was the first commercially available medium contained 2.5–10% chondroitin sulphate [27]. *In vitro* and *in vivo* efficacy of

K-Sol storage medium for high level corneal endothelial viability has been demonstrated in numerous studies. Some studies did not recognize any reduction in endothelial survival in corneas stored for 2–3 days in M–K medium or in 1–2 weeks in K-Sol medium [28]. Clinical studies showed good endothelial cell preservation and no difference between the corneas stored in M–K medium for 2–3 days and K-Sol medium for 1–2 weeks. However, K-Sol medium is no longer commercially available due to problems with tissue contamination with Propionibacterium acnes, first noted in 1988, and it was not reintroduced again [29].

A new formula for chondroitin sulphate corneal storage medium (CSM) was then developed for intermediate-term storage at 4°C and long-term storage in 37°C [30]. The superior efficiency of CSM for prolonging endothelial cell viability over K-Sol was demonstrated in various *in vitro* studies—the efficiency of CSM was comparable with K-Sol medium for storage in 4°C for 7–10 days. Further storage for 14–20 days showed significantly higher endothelial cell damage in corneas stored in K-Sol than in CSM. No significant difference in endothelial cell density after corneal transplantation (3, 6, 9 and 12 months after grafting) was found in paired corneas stored in K-Sol or CSM medium for 8–97 hours [31].

Later developments in storage media based on chondroitin sulphate-containing formulae, include Optisol and Dexsol. Both contain chondroitin sulphate (Optisol 2.5% and Dexsol 1.5%), 1% dextran, gentamicin, sodium pyruvate, nonessential amino acids and additional antioxidants. Optisol has also ATP precursors, ascorbic acid and vitamin B_{12}. Both showed superiority to M–K medium, K-Sol and CMS and are commercially available at the moment [32–34].

Problems with donor availability and timing of surgery in relation to need and indication for corneal grafting have led to developments for long-term corneal preservation. Organ culture is a method for long-term corneal preservation. This technique was originally introduced by Doughman in 1976. He used a 20 ml Petri dish, which contained organ culture medium for storage [35]. The medium had to be exchanged three times per week, which increased the possibility of microbial contamination. Therefore, a closed system—the Minnesota system—was introduced [36]. This system uses medium containing 1.35% chondroitin sulphate, 10% fetal calf serum, Eagle's tissue culture medium, gentamicin, HEPES, nonessential amino acids and antioxidant.

The globe is washed with disinfectant solution, rinsed for 1 minute in saline and then flushed with saline. A limbal swab is taken for microbiological culture. The cornea is excised from the globe and placed in a Petri dish with 15 ml of medium. The cornea stays in the Petri dish for 2–3 days in 34°C in an incubator in the presence of 5% CO_2. After this period of time, the cornea is transferred to 130 ml of organ culture medium in a sterile sealed bottle and maintained at 34°C. Seven days after incubation in organ culture, 10 ml of medium is removed from the bottle and cultured for bacterial and fungal infection. If no growth is detected after 10 days and the medium in the closed bottle is clear, the system is sterile and the cornea can be utilized for transplantation. Corneas prepared in this manner can be stored up to 35 days [37].

The advantage of this technique is long storage time, which allows detection and possibly elimination of infection agents. The major disadvantage is the technical complexity and special equipment needed for this type of corneal preservation.

Future Developments

A constant demand for corneal tissue has led to research in tissue engineering which currently is in a very promising position. The bioengineered ocular surface tissue replacement consisting of (presumed) human corneal epithelial stem cells in a cross-linked fibrin gel can be used for potential transplantation and provides the potential for a totally autologous bioengineered replacement tissue [38–40] (see also Chapter 13). In addition, the standard use of organ cultured corneas allows for the possibility of manipulations such as coating donor corneas with antibodies or genetic manipulation (see Chapter 10). *In vitro* modifications of the donor cornea with gene transfer can be an important advance to modulate the functions of endothelial cells and to protect them from immune attack [41]. Currently adenovirus transfer of IL-10 or CTLA-4 has the potential to modulate immunological rejection in animal models, which is still the major cause of corneal graft failure [42–44] (see Chapter 10).

References

1. Zirm E. *Eine erfolgreich totale Keratoplastik*. *Arch Ophthalmol* 1906; 64: 580.
2. Filatov VP. Transplantation of the cornea. *Arch Ophthalmol* 1935; 13: 321.
3. Farge EJ. Eye banking: 1944 to the present. *Surv Ophthalmol* 1989; 33(4): 260.
4. Wilson SE and Bourne WM. Corneal preservation for penetrating keratoplasty. In: Kaufman HE, Barron BA and McDonald MB, *The Cornea*. Butterworth-Heinemann, Boston, 1998; 781.

5. Stocker FW. The endothelium of the cornea and its clinical implications. *Trans Am Ophthalmol Soc* 1953; 51: 669.
6. Capella JA, Kaufman HE and Robbins JE. Preservation of viable corneal tissue. *Arch Ophthalmol* 1965; 74: 669.
7. McCarey BE, Meyer RF and Kaufman HE. Improved corneal storage for penetrating keratoplasties in humans. *Ann Ophthalmol* 1976; 8(12): 1488, 1495.
8. Mizukawa T and Manabe R. Recent advances in keratoplasty with special reference to the advantages of liquid preservation. *Nippon Ganka Kiyo* 1968; 19: 1310.
9. McGinn P. Regulatory matters: new Europe-wide law to regulate tissue implants. *ESCRS Eurotimes* 2002; 7: 35.
10. Shiuey Y and Moshirfar M. Use of infant donor tissue for endokeratoplasty. *J Cataract Refract Surg* 2001; 27(12): 1915.
11. Lane SS, Mizener MW, Dubbel PA, Mindrup EA, Wick AA, Doughman DJ and Holland EJ. Whole globe enucleation versus *in situ* corneal excision: a study of tissue trauma and contamination. *Cornea* 1994; 13(4): 305.
12. Vannas S. Excision of the donor cornea instead of enucleation. *Invest Ophthalmol* 1975; 14(4): 293.
13. Stocker FW, King EH, Lucas DO and Georgiade N. A comparison of two different staining methods for evaluating corneal endothelial viability. *Arch Ophthalmol* 1966; 76: 1966.
14. Kuming BS. The assessment of endothelial viability. *South Afr Med J* 1969; 43: 1083.
15. Kolb MJ and Bourne WM. Supravital fluorescent staining of the corneal endothelium with acridine orange and ethidium bromide. *Curr Eye Res* 1986; 5: 485.
16. Harris JE and Nordquist LT. The hydration of the cornea. I. Transport water from the cornea. *Am J Ophthalmol* 1955; 40: 100.
17. Schaeffer EM. Ultrastructural changes in moist chamber corneas. *Invest Ophthalmol* 1963; 2: 272.
18. Hoefle FB, Maurice DM and Sibley RC. Human corneal donor material. *Arch Ophthalmol* 1970; 84: 741.
19. Means TL, Geroski DH and Hadley A. Viability of human corneal endothelium following Optisol-GS storage. *Arch Ophthalmol* 1995; 113: 805.
20. Taylor MJ. Clinical cryobiology of tissues: preservation of corneas. *Cryobiology* 1986; 23(4): 323.
21. O'Neill P, Mueller FO and Trevor-Roper PD. On the preservation of corneae at –196°C for full-thickness homografts in man and dog. *Br J Ophthalmol* 1967; 51: 13.
22. Delbosc B, Herve P, Carbillet JP and Montard M. Corneal cryopreservation in man: a proposal for an original technic. *J Fr Ophtalmol* 1984; 7(4): 321.
23. Canals M, Costa J, Potau JM, Merindano MD, Pita D and Ruano D. Long-term cryopreservation of human donor corneas. *Eur J Ophthalmol* 1996; 6(3): 234.
24. Brunette I, Le Francois M, Tremblay MC and Guertin MC. Corneal transplant tolerance of cryopreservation. *Cornea* 2001; 20(6): 590.
25. Van Horn DL, Schultz RO and Edelhauser HF. Corneal cryopreservation: alterations in endothelial intercellular spaces. *Am J Ophthalmol* 1969; 68(3): 454.
26. Moll AC, Van Rij G, Beekhuis WH, Reneradel de Lavalette JH, Hermans J, Pels E and Rinkel-van Driel E. Effect of donor cornea preservation in tissue culture and in

McCarey–Kaufmann medium on corneal graft rejection and visual acuity. *Doc Ophthalmol* 1991; 78(3–4): 273.

27. Kaufman HE,Varnell ED and Kaufman S. Chondroitin sulphate in a new cornea preservation medium. *Am J Ophthalmol* 1984; 98: 112.
28. Busin M,Yau C,Avni I and Kaufman HE. Comparison of K-Sol and M–K medium for cornea storage: results of penetrating keratoplasty in rabbits. *Br J Ophthalmol* 1986; 70: 860.
29. Sieck EA, Enzenauer RW, Cornell M and Butler C. Contamination of K-Sol corneal storage with *Propionibacterium acnes*. *Arch Ophthalmol* 1989; 107: 1023.
30. Lass JH, Reinhart WJ, Skelnik *et al.* An *in vitro* and clinical comparison of corneal storage with chondroitin sulphate corneal storage medium with or without dextran. *Ophthalmology* 1990; 97: 96.
31. Lass JH, Reinhart WJ, Bruner WE *et al.* Comparison of corneal storage in K-Sol and chondroitin sulphate corneal storage medium in human corneal transplantation. *Ophthalmology* 1989; 96: 688.
32. Frueh BE and Bohnke M. Prospective, randomized clinical evaluation of Optisol vs organ culture corneal storage media. *Arch Ophthalmol* 2000; 118(6): 757.
33. Lass JH, Bourne WM, Musch DC, Sugar A, Gordon JF, Reinhart WJ, Meyer RF, Patel DI, Bruner WE, Cano DB, *et al.* A randomized, prospective, double-masked clinical trial of Optisol vs DexSol corneal storage media. *Arch Ophthalmol* 1992; 110(10): 1404.
34. Yap C,Wong AM, Naor J and Rootman DS. Corneal temperature reversal after storage in Chen medium compared with Optisol GS. *Cornea* 2001; 20(5): 501.
35. Doughman DJ, Harris JE and Schmitt MK. Penetrating keratoplasty using 37°C organ cultured cornea. *Trans Am Acad Ophthalmol Otolarynol* 1976; 81: 778.
36. Cowden JW. Careful Michigan procedures screen donor eyes for any disease. *Mich Med* 1979 ; 78(11): 195.
37. Ehlers H, Ehlers N and Hjortdal JO. Corneal transplantation with donor tissue kept in organ culture for 7 weeks. *Acta Ophthalmol Scand* 1999; 77(3): 277.
38. Ferber D. Tissue engineering. Growing human corneas in the lab. *Science* 1999; 286(5447): 2051, 2053.
39. Han B, Schwab IR, Madsen TK and Isseroff RR. A fibrin-based bioengineered ocular surface with human corneal epithelial stem cells. *Cornea* 2002; 21(5): 505.
40. Germain L,Auger FA, Grandbois E, Guignard R, Giasson M, Boisjoly H and Guerin SL. Reconstructed human cornea produced in vitro by tissue engineering. *Pathobiology* 1999; 67(3): 140.
41. Pleyer U, Groth D, Hinz B, Keil O, Bertelmann E, Rieck P and Reszka R. Efficiency and toxicity of liposome-mediated gene transfer to corneal endothelial cells. *Exp Eye Res* 2001; 73(1): 1.
42. Klebe S, Sykes PJ, Coster DJ, Bloom DC and Williams KA. Gene transfer to ovine corneal endothelium. *Clin Exp Ophthalmol* 2001; 29(5): 316.
43. Klebe S, Sykes PJ, Coster DJ, Krishnan R and Williams KA. Prolongation of sheep corneal allograft survival by *ex vivo* transfer of the gene encoding interleukin-10. *Transplantation* 2001; 71(9): 1214.
44. Comer RM, King WJ, Ardjomand N, Theoharis S, George AJ and Larkin DF. Effect of administration of CTLA4-Ig as protein or cDNA on corneal allograft survival. *Invest Ophthalmol Vis Sci* 2002; 43(4): 1095.

5

MHC Antigens, Tissue Typing and Blood Group Matching in Corneal Transplantation

Introduction

Early studies in transplantation, mostly in the skin, pointed clearly towards genetic regulation of graft acceptance, in both humans and mice. The key to the discovery of the MHC was the use of inbred strains of mice which after many rounds of sibling matings (usually about 20) are syngeneic, i.e. homozygous at every chromosome pair for all the different alleles of any given protein while the corresponding "wild type" mice are allogeneic. Most of the large animals used for corneal grafting (see Chapter 8) are outbred and therefore allogeneic when grafting within species.

Skin grafts from nonsyngeneic mice were seen to undergo rapid rejection and by breeding several strains of congenic mice this was shown to be due to differences (polymorphisms) at a restricted genetic region, previously known as polymorphic blood group Antigen II and later histocompatibility-2 or H-2. Further studies showed that this region contained several genes (see Figure 5.1A), termed the major histocompatibility complex (MHC), and that both genes in any allelic pair of chromosomes are expressed, i.e. they are codominant. In addition, studies on antibody responses to different antigens in mice pointed to the existence of immune response (Ir) genes which were found to be located within the MHC regions, were also highly polymorphic, and were allelically selective in their capacity to bind different

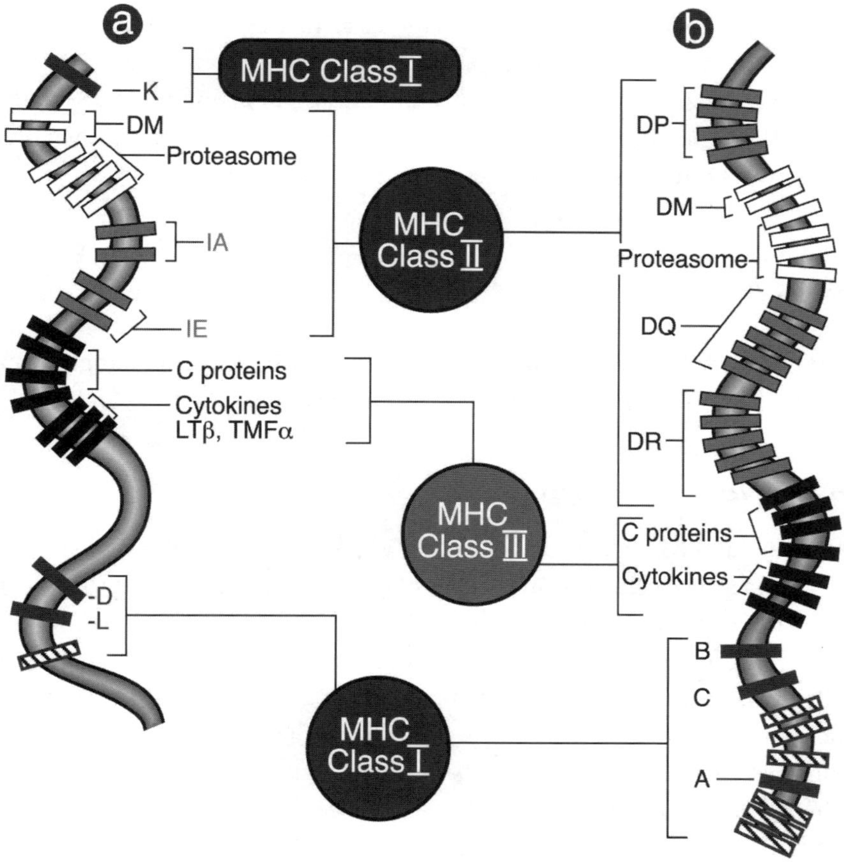

Figure 5.1 Diagram of HLA locus. (**A**) Mouse H-2 region; (**B**) human HLA region.

antigenic peptides leading to either a weak or strong antibody response. Presentation of peptide to T cells to provide help to B cells has since been shown to be the underlying mechanism.

Identification of the homologous system in humans came from serological studies of patients who had had blood transfusions or organ transplants as a result of which they were frequently observed to develop lytic antibodies to white blood cells in the presence of complement. From this it was clear that these sera recognised antigens on the white blood cells, known as human leukocyte antigens (HLA), for which there were three major or Class I genes, HLA-A, -B and -C, and a later set known as HLA-D-related or HLA-DR. Since then the science of MHC genes has expanded to include many other genes and molecular techniques have now been applied to identify the >1300 different allotypes identified for the human MHC gene set [1].

In these experiments, it soon became clear that not all skin graft experiments ran true to the MHC paradigm and that other genes were also involved. These are known as the minor histocompatibility genes or the non-MHC genes and most of these show much lower degrees of polymorphism compared to MHC antigens.

MHC Antigens

In humans, MHC antigens are known as human leukocyte antigens and in mice and rats they are termed H-2 antigens.

Human leukocyte antigens

Fischer and Mayr have defined HLA as a set of glycoproteins which take up peptides intracellularly and become ligands for immune receptors when they are expressed on the cell surface [2]. This definition, while not describing the essential nature of these proteins, i.e. their high degree of polymorphism which underlies individual characteristics, does highlight their most important function, i.e. that they are central to the adaptive immune response and are the basis for rejection of solid organ grafts whether by the direct or the indirect route (see Chapter 6).

MHC Class I molecules are composed of a heavy α chain and a light β chain. The β chain binds noncovalently to the α chain and has no direct link to the cell surface. The three-dimensional conformation of the MHC Class I molecule comprises a peptide binding groove, an immunoglobulin-like domain, a transmembrane region and a cytoplasmic domain (Figure 5.2). The MHC encoded polymorphic region resides in the heavy chain and it is here that the great variation in the amino acid sequence determines the haplotype (i.e. the full set of MHC allotypes) of the individual and thus the affinity each specific MHC molecule has for different peptides. The peptide binding groove is formed by two sequences of about 90 amino acids long at the N terminus of the molecule, each termed $\alpha 1$ and $\alpha 2$ segments; the $\alpha 3$ segment binds to the β segment in the region of the Ig-like domain. Presentation of allopeptide (and other foreign peptides) by the indirect route of antigen presentation occurs by the binding of processed nine-mer peptides to the groove; in contrast presentation of alloantigen (i.e. the intact MHC molecule) by the direct route does not involve processing of the alloantigen and it is thought that such alloantigens may either have "empty"

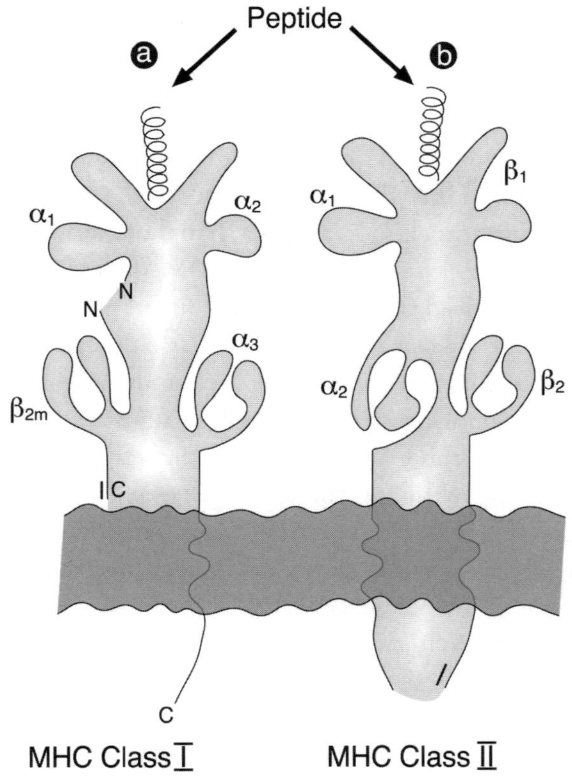

Figure 5.2 Diagrams of HLA molecules. (**A**) Human MHC molecule class I; (**B**) human MHC molecule class II.

grooves or may contain self peptides. MHC Class I molecules present peptide preferentially to CD8+ T cells and the α3 constant region is responsible for binding to CD8 antigen on T cells.

MHC Class II molecules are composed of two polypeptides, an α chain and a β chain held together in a noncovalent interaction. The two proteins form a peptide-binding groove as for the MHC Class I. Both chains are polymorphic and encoded by different regions of the MHC, but otherwise have many similarities to Class I molecules with an Ig-like domain, a transmembrane region and a cytoplasmic domain (Figure 5.2B). The peptide binding region is formed by the α1 and β1 regions of the α and β molecules respectively, using α helices and β strands to form the walls and floor of the grooves as for the two α1 sequences of the Class I molecule. The α2 and β2 regions are relatively constant and a portion of the β2 molecule binds the CD4 molecule on T cells.

Organization of HLA on the human genome

The MHC in humans maps to the short arm of chromosome 6. In addition to the well known antigens such as HLA-A, -B, -C and -D (P, Q and R) there are many other genes found in this region some belonging to the MHC. These include HLA-E, -F, -G, -H and -J, the complement genes (MHC Class III), heat shock protein genes, lymphotoxins a and b, and the proteasome genes TAP-1 and -2 and HLA-DM (Figure 5.1B). Many of these are directly involved in immunological functions including antigen processing, while the role of others is less clear although they may have unexpected roles such as the recently proposed immunoregulatory role for HLA-G [3]. The nonpolymorpic gene HLA-H is involved in iron metabolism and mutations in this gene cause haemochromatosis. One suggestion for the role of the many nonpolymorphic genes and pseudogenes in the MHC region is to provide a nucleotide resource for gene conversion within the MHC Class I and II genes, an efficient mechanism for increasing polymorphism in the MHC.

As indicated above, each gene has many allotypes and extensive refinement of the genetic differences between allotypes has been achieved using molecular techniques. Much of this information is now available through electronic databases and represents a rich research resource. In practical terms, matching for organ transplantation has taken on a new perspective in that complete molecular matching is rarely possible except between identical twins. In addition, it is now recognised that some allelic differences may be less deleterious for graft acceptance than others and thus the strategy of identifying favourable versus unfavourable MHC differences in matching host and donor for solid organ transplantation is now the philosophy of most transplantation centres.

Interesting differences exist in heterozygous expression of MHC Class I and Class II in humans. For MHC Class I, each cell may express up to six different alleles (two each of HLA-A, -B and -C) but for MHC Class II, due to the fact that each individual may express two different β chains for each α chain and also because each allele of the α chain may bind to either or both the β alleles, it is possible for an MHC Class II positive cell to express between 10 and 20 different MHC molecules simultaneously. This greatly increases the number of possible CD4+ T cell interactions each cell may have and explains in part why some sets of allelic differences may induce less alloreactivity than others since it also depends somewhat on the clonal frequency of the corresponding set of host T cell receptors.

Murine H-2 antigens

Murine H-2 antigens are also segregated into MHC Class I, MHC Class II and complement genes. There are three MHC Class I genes, namely K, D and L and two MHC class II genes designated I-A and I-E (Figure 5.1A). Human haplotypes (i.e. the set of allotypes that characterize any one individual) are described as numerals while murine haplotypes use letters. Since most murine haplotypes represent inbred homozygous states a typical murine haplotype would thus be H-2K^d, I-A^d, I-E^d, D^d, L^d. The H-2K and D loci are considered to be the most important for direct alloantigen graft rejection.

The ordered sequence of genes on the murine MHC on chromosome 17 is slightly different from the human MHC on chromosome 6 (see Figure 5.1). In addition, the I-A region actually codes for the α and β chains of the I-A molecule as well as the α chain of the I-E molecule, while the I-E region codes for the β chain of I-E.

Minor Histocompatibility Antigens

Minor antigens were identified from genetic disparities in mouse skin grafting experiments which could not be explained by MHC genes. Minor H antigens participate in the alloreactive response by virtue of polymorphic differences but their effect is masked by the strong MHC alloresponse. Minor antigens are presented as peptides on MHC antigens via the indirect pathway and they are therefore recognized when MHC alleles are shared between host and donor [4]. In view of the fact that several MHC Class I and Class II genes are involved in the direct alloresponse, chance predicts that some of these alleles may be shared, thus facilitating presentation of the minor antigens [5]. Indirect minor antigen allopresentation is considered to form the immunological basis of one component of chronic immune rejection.

Most minor H genes are unidentified or characterised, and most have low levels of polymorphism, often being no more than a single amino acid difference [5]. However, information on minor antigens is accumulating. Some are related to the male H-Y antigen and others to antigens expressed on haematopoietic cells. Two more recently described genes in the mouse are the Uty and the SMCY genes which are also male specific genes present in the mouse, and an autosomal gene of the H-13 allele in the mouse [4].

Tissue Typing and HLA Matching

Solid organ vascularized grafts are usually tissue typed for compatibility using a range of tests including cross matching (for blood group antibodies), HLA typing and applying functional tests such as the mixed leukocyte reaction (MLR) test and cytotoxicity testing. Sensitization to allografts is tested for by determining alloantibody levels and most recently by measuring T cell cytokine responses to alloantigen for instance by ELISA or in an ELISPOT assay (see below).

The MLR

The allogeneic MLR is a measure of potential direct alloreactivity of host lymphocytes to donor antigen. In human MLR, peripheral blood mononuclear cells from both the donor and host are cultured together *in vitro* for 3–7 days and the proliferative potential of the host and/or donor leukocytes is measured by incorporation of radioactive thymidine. In rodents, lymph node or spleen cells are used. The assay is based on the expression and presentation of intact MHC antigens, predominantly MHC Class II antigens [6], on donor antigen-presenting cells to host alloreactive T cells. Cells responding to MHC Class II antigens are CD4+ T cells while cells responding to MHC Class I antigen are CD8+ T cells and are the main mediators of the cytotoxicity assay (cytotoxic lymphocytes, CTLs; see below). CD4+ T cells induced to proliferate in an MLR assay will produce an accelerated response (2–3 days) if harvested and rechallenged with the same MHC Class II antigen in a second MLR. The separation of responder cells (see below) into MHC Class I-CD8 and MHC Class II-CD4 is not absolute: cytotoxic CD4+ T cells may be induced and some CD8+ T cells produce a panel of cytokines similar to Th1 cells.

Two tests are described: the one-way and the two-way MLR. In the one-way MLR, proliferation of donor T lymphocytes and antigen presenting cells is inhibited by prior irradiation sufficient to prevent cell division but not to kill the cells. Alternatively, proliferation of donor APCs can be inhibited by use of drugs such as mitomycin C. Donor cells so treated are described as stimulators. In the one way assay only host T cells can respond to donor antigen (known as responders) and the results can be interpreted as an indication of direct allosensitivity. In the two-way assay no inhibition of proliferation is induced, and both donor and host T cells can respond. This test is used to determine the risk of graft versus host disease which is presumed to be due to chimerism and proliferation of donor cells responding to host antigen.

The one-way MLR is used to dissect out MHC Class I and II differences between potential donor and host combinations. Each cell in the MLR responds to a single alloantigen and thus if there are many allelic differences the response is correspondingly stronger. In addition, since each APC expresses several different MHC antigens simultaneously due to codominance of MHC genes (see above), many T cells of differing T cell receptor (TCR) specificity may be induced by the same APC. The assay is sufficiently sensitive to identify single point mutations in MHC genes at the molecular level but is labour- and time-intensive.

Cytotoxicity assay

CTLs bind preferentially to cells expressing high levels of MHC Class I. This includes professional antigen-presenting cells, but also many non-antigen-presenting cells especially if their MHC antigens have been upregulated by inflammatory stimuli, e.g. after viral infection. CTLs bind to MHC Class I–expressing cells due to their affinity via the CD8 molecule for the nonpolymorhpic region of the Class I molecule, while the polymorphic regions bind directly to the TCR (direct allorecognition) or via host MHC-allopeptide complexes (indirect allorecognition; see Chapter 6). Donor allografts, especially skin, upregulate their complement of MHC and are thus liable to acute rejection. This is mediated via direct killing of the graft cells via granule exocytosis-dependent (perforin, granzyme, etc.) and -independent (Fas; FasL) mechanisms.

CTLs generated in an MLR or directly harvested from blood and lymphoid organs can be tested in a cytotoxicity assay using target cells, labelled with Cr^{51}, which are induced to express high levels of MHC Class I. As for the MLR, depending on the number of mismatches at the Class I loci, increased levels of cytolysis will occur and thus can be quantitated by determining the amount of Cr^{51} released. CTL testing in patients after corneal graft has shown that sensitization on MHC class I antigens can occur [7, 8].

Tests of allosensitization

Tests of allosensitization are relatively less commonly performed but may be of value particularly in cases of regrafting. Historically, this is usually tested indirectly by measuring alloantibody responses, which are presumed to be the result of activated T cell help for B cells but correlation with graft outcome is not strong. In addition, while the MLR is useful for determining the "alloreactivity" of a naïve host to a potential donor, it has limited value in assessing the level of "allosensitization" of the host, i.e. the memory cell response after grafting.

In a recent study of the allogeneic delayed hypersensitivity response in renal allograft patients, which utilized a *trans vivo* method of subcutanoeaus injecton of human peripheral blood monocytes in mice together with alloantigen, it was shown that up to 50% of patients display sensitized T cells to the allograft [9]. This was considerably higher than the incidence of alloantibodies to the graft in the same group of patients. Interestingly, there was also no correlation with the number of HLA mismatches between the donor–host pairs (up to six mismathces tested), nor with clinical outcome. Since many of these patients were treated with immunosuppressants, the data suggested that the effect of these drugs is on the effector stage of the alloimmune response and not on sensitization.

Release of cytokines by T cells is a measure of antigen activation and thus of prior sensitization to antigen. Examination of peripheral blood T cells for intracellular cytokine by flow cytometry or for bulk cytokine production *in vitro* by ELISA has been performed but may not be sufficiently discriminatory as yet. Recent use of the ELISPOT assay to determine cytokine production at the single cell level was shown to correlate with the clinical outcome of graft acceptance [10]. In this assay, tissue culture plates were coated with capture antibody to a range of cytokines, incubated with responder T cells and activated by donor stimulator cells. Release of cytokine by individual cells was then assayed by using a second anticytokine antibody labelled with a detector molecule. Graft rejection episodes appeared to correlate with the level of IFN-γ-secreting responder T lymphocytes.

Blood group antigens

Although much attention has been paid to the MHC antigens in solid organ transplantation, the ABO blood group antigenic system is a considerably stronger barrier to transplantation success than the HLA and any patient being considered for solid organ vascularized grafting is initially cross-matched for blood group antigens. Very few ABO-incompatible solid organ grafts have been successfully accepted (for review see Ref. 11).

Interestingly, the HLA barrier is stronger for bone marrow grafts than the ABO system.

The ABO system is important since humans have "natural" antibodies against those ABO(H) antigens which are not present in the individual and thus can induce acute or hyperacute rejection as in xenografts. It is believed that as for xenoantibodies, ABO blood group antibodies develop through cross-reactivity with microbial antigens during colonization of the gut in early childhood (see Chapter 7).

ABO antigens are glycosphingolipids. The core O antigen is a glycan which is present in all individuals and thus induces tolerance, i.e. no anti-O antibodies exist. The A and B antigens are sugar-based moieties which are added to the core O antigen. There are three common alleles of the glycosyl trasferase enzyme, of which the A allele transfers a N-acetylgalactosamine residue, the B allele transfers a galactose moiety, and the O allele has no activity. Thus there are four allelic variants of ABO antigens: O (OO), A (AA, AO), B (BB, BO) and AB (A, B), in which the various subsets of individuals have no determinant (O, OO), the N-acetylgalactosamine determinant (AA, AO), the galactose determinant (BB, BO) or both the N-acetylgalactosamine and the galactosamine antigenic determinants (AB) added to the O glycan core. Minor modifications to the core antigen can also be made by other glycosyltrasferases, which add fucosyl residues to the sugar chain, and O antigens which have been so modified are known as H antigens, thus termed the ABO(H) antigen blood group system. The fucosyl residue is present in nearly all individuals and sometimes more than one is added to the core antigen, thus generating diversity in what is known as the Lewis antigen, important as ligands for the E- and P-selectin adhesion molecules.

ABO blood group antigens are expressed on many tissues in addition to red cells. Variants of the A, B and H chains have been described and the four different Gal-GlucNac chains are variably expressed in different tissues [11]; for instance, kidney tissue contains more type 4 chain than other tissues. In addition, subgroup A1 individuals express a greater total number of blood group antigens in tissues than A2, thus making it possible to transplant ABH (A2) grafts more readily. Blood group antigens in tissues are preferentially expressed on vascular endothelium but are also found on parenchymal cells although expression is variable, e.g. high on glomeruli but low on kidney tubules. They are absent on hepatocytes but present on bile duct epithelium.

Because the early experience with ABH incompatible grafts was universal rejection, cross-matched recipients were considered to be mandatory. However, with immunosuppression and antibody depletion, some ABH incompatible grafts can survive despite the fact that antibodies reappear after some weeks and this acceptance of the incompatible grafts is termed accommodation (see Chapter 7). Steady progress in grafting vascularized ABO(H)-incompatible grafts is being made, with careful selection of donor/recipient pairs and the use of strong immunosuppressive regimes.

Corneal transplantation and MHC matching

Corneal grafts in humans are usually performed without tissue matching. The one-year survival rate for corneal allografts is excellent [12], and the three- and five-year outcomes, although not as good as other solid organ grafts, are comparable [13] (see also Chapter 6). Late graft failure in most tissues is considered to be due to chronic rejection, although tissue-dependent causes may also contribute to the overall late failure rates in all grafts [14].

Controversy exists over whether MHC matching has any role in promoting corneal graft success. Many factors contribute to success or failure, including loosening of sutures (induction of innate immunity) and corneal vascularization rather than MHC mismatching [15]. Corneas are categorized on the basis of high or low risk. There is a consensus that HLA matching does not confer a significant advantage on low risk grafts and this is supported by a large prospective randomized study [12]. However, some believe that HLA matching in high risk grafts, such as second or third time regrafts, or grafts to highly vascularized recipient beds, is beneficial [16].

Tissue typing and matching for MHC antigens in vascularized organs is considered to reduce the amount of direct alloantigen recognition and acute rejection of grafts. However, the normal corneal endothelium (the main target of allorecognition) does not constitutively express significant levels of MHC Class I and thus direct allorecognition and MHC Class I: CD8+ T cell–mediated cytotoxic responses are considered not to be prominent in corneal graft rejection (see Chapter 6). Therefore matching for MHC Class I would seem from first principles to be unnecessary. However, despite initial reports there is evidence that matching in certain circumstances promotes better graft survival rates especially after high risk grafting [13]. Theoretically it is possible that there might be upregulation of MHC Class I on corneal parenchymal cells and also on the now recognized passenger leukocytes in the donor graft [17, 18] induced by local cytokine production from host cells in the high risk vascularized bed. A beneficial effect of HLA matching thus might be explained by minimizing direct and indirect allopresentation of this upregulated MHC class I antigen.

More controversial still is the question of matching for MHC Class II antigen in corneal allografting. Initial studies suggested that mismatching at the MHC Class II loci might be beneficial for eventual graft outcome [19]. While a positive benefit might be difficult to show, it is theoretically possible that certain MHC mismatches may be more favourable for graft acceptance than others and, combined with the multitude of other factors impinging on survival rate of corneal grafts, a chance overall benefit might emerge from some statistical analysis [20]. However, a beneficial effect from mismatching at the Class II loci was not observed in other large studies of corneal graft, and indeed the opposite appeared to be the case [21]. Some of the controversy over differences in results has been attributed to insensitivity of the typing methods used for evaluating Class II matching.

A recent study has provided valuable insight into the role of HLA typing using modern molecular techniques for analysis of MHC antigens. In a retrospective analysis of the number of matches between donor and recipient it was shown that two or more matches at the HLA A locus but not the HLA B locus reduced the incidence of rejection episodes; similarly, in a subset of high risk grafts with vascularized corneal recipient beds, it was found that two or more matches on HLA DRB1 reduced the risk of rejection [16]. Despite the authors' stated reservations regarding aspects of the study such as the low numbers of cases studied and differences in some case control groups, the conclusions regarding the above data seem sound. In particular, the widespread use of organ culture for corneas prior to grafting allows time for adequate molecular typing of grafts and at least for high risk cases, HLA matching on both Class I and Class II would seem to be a valuable procedure.

Corneal grafting and ABO

Vascularized solid organ grafts are rarely accepted across ABO blood group barriers. Despite this corneal grafts are usually performed without any level of matching, be it HLA or ABO blood group matching. At least for high risk grafts into vascularized recipient beds it might seem prudent to match for blood group [22]. There is some supportive clinical evidence. A retrospective study of high risk vs low risk grafts indicated that the risk of rejection was increased in the absence of ABO compatibility [23], although a previous study could not find any beneficial effect of matching for ABO [24]. However, the CCTS in its prospective study found supportive evidence for ABO matching in prolonging graft survival [12].

Blood group antigens are thought to be present only on epithelial cells in normal corneas [25], although there is some indirect evidence that they may also be present on the corneal endothelium [26]. In diseased corneas ABO antigens are expressed at high levels in stromal keratoctyes and endothelial cells and they have been postulated to play a role in graft rejection in high risk corneas [27]. How this might occur is not clear since ABO expression on donor cornea rather than the host is the presumed target of host natural antibodies and evidence for high levels of ABO antigens on corneal endothelium is not available. No evidence for increased risk was found in patients who might have been prior sensitized via blood transfusion or pregnancy [28]. In addition, the tempo of rejection is such that acute rejection via humoral mechanisms is not likely, although it is possible that such mechanisms could account for rare cases of unexplained "primary" graft failure. Interestingly, compatibility of Lewis antigen has been found to be valuable in outcomes of nonvascularized corneal grafts but not high risk vascularized grafts [29]. Further study of blood group antigen expression on corneal tissue is warranted.

Conclusion

Corneal graft rejection is considered to occur predominantly by the indirect allorecognition route. Both the low total dose of alloantigen and absence of vessels contribute to the low allogenicity of corneal allografts, which thus have a high rate of acceptance after one year even for full HLA mismatches. However, the long-term outcomes (five years and more) are poor and are particularly so in high risk grafts, e.g. in a vascularized recipient bed or a regraft after previous graft rejection. Under these circumstances the evidence for a beneficial effect for HLA matching on both Class I and class II is strong and probably reflects increased alloantigen presentation by the indirect route although the possibility for some direct allopresentation is also present. Modern molecular techniques of HLA matching can provide a quantitative prognosis for good and not as good matching outcomes. Importantly, ABO(H) blood group matching in high risk grafting should be considered.

References

1. Robinson J and Marsh SG. The IMGT/HLA sequence database. *Rev Immunogenet* 2000; 2(4): 518.
2. Fischer GF and Mayr WR. Molecular genetics of the HLA complex. *Wien Klin Wochenschr* 2001; 113(20–21): 814.
3. Rouas-Freiss N *et al.* HLA-G in transplantation: a relevant molecule for inhibition of graft rejection? *Am J Transplant* 2003; 3(1): 11.
4. Simpson E *et al.* Minor H antigens: genes and peptides. *Transpl Immunol* 2002; 10(2–3): 115.
5. Engelhard VH, Brickner AG and Zarling AL. Insights into antigen processing gained by direct analysis of the naturally processed class I MHC associated peptide repertoire. *Mol Immunol* 2002; 39(3–4): 127.
6. Steinman RM and Inaba K. Stimulation of the primary mixed leukocyte reaction. *Crit Rev Immunol* 1985; 5(4): 331.
7. Hahn AB *et al.* The association of lymphocytotoxic antibodies with corneal allograft rejection in high risk patients: The Collaborative Corneal Transplantation Studies Research Group. *Transplantation* 1995; 59(1): 21.
8. Roelen DL *et al.* The presence of activated donor HLA class I-reactive T lymphocytes is associated with rejection of corneal grafts. *Transplantation* 1995; 59(7): 1039.
9. Pelletier RP *et al.* High incidence of donor-reactive delayed-type hypersensitivity reactivity in transplant patients. *Am J Transplant* 2002; 2(10): 926.
10. Heeger PS *et al.* Pretransplant frequency of donor-specific, IFN-gamma-producing lymphocytes is a manifestation of immunologic memory and correlates with the risk of posttransplant rejection episodes. *J Immunol* 1999; 163(4): 2267.
11. Rydberg L. ABO-incompatibility in solid organ transplantation. *Transfus Med* 2001; 11(4): 325.
12. The collaborative corneal transplantation studies (CCTS): Effectiveness of histocompatibility matching in high-risk corneal transplantation. The Collaborative Corneal Transplantation Studies Research Group. *Arch Ophthalmol* 1992; 110(10): 1392.
13. Williams KA *et al.* How successful is corneal transplantation? A report from the Australian Corneal Graft Register. *Eye* 1995; 9(Pt 2): 219.
14. Gourishankar S and Halloran PF. Late deterioration of organ transplants: a problem in injury and homeostasis. *Curr Opin Immunol* 2002; 14(5): 576.
15. Jonas JB, Rank RM and Budde WM. Immunologic graft reactions after allogenic penetrating keratoplasty. *Am J Ophthalmol* 2002; 133(4): 437.
16. Bartels MC *et al.* Influence of HLA-A, HLA-B, and HLA-DR matching on rejection of random corneal grafts using corneal tissue for retrospective DNA HLA typing. *Br J Ophthalmol* 2001; 85(11): 1341.
17. Brissette-Storkus CS *et al.* Identification of a novel macrophage population in the normal mouse corneal stroma. *Invest Ophthalmol Vis Sci* 2002; 43(7): 2264.
18. Liu Y *et al.* Draining lymph nodes of corneal transplant hosts exhibit evidence for donor major histocompatibility complex (MHC) class II-positive dendritic cells derived from MHC class II-negative grafts. *J Exp Med* 2002; 195(2): 259.
19. Vail A *et al.* Conclusions of the corneal transplant follow up study: collaborating surgeons. *Br J Ophthalmol* 1997; 81(8): 631.

20. Claas FH *et al.* Future HLA matching strategies in clinical transplantation. *Dev Ophthalmol* 2003; 36: 62.
21. Volker-Dieben HJ *et al.* Beneficial effect of HLA-DR matching on the survival of corneal allografts. *Transplantation* 2000; 70(4): 640.
22. Borderie VM *et al.* ABO antigen blood-group compatibility in corneal transplantation. *Cornea* 1997; 16(1): 1
23. Inoue K and Tsuru T. ABO antigen blood-group compatibility and allograft rejection in corneal transplantation. *Acta Ophthalmol Scand* 1999; 77(5): 495.
24. Batchelor JR *et al.* HLA matching and corneal grafting. *Lancet* 1976; 1(7959): 551.
25. Treseler PA, Foulks GN and Sanfilippo F. Expression of ABO blood group, hematopoietic, and other cell-specific antigens by cells in the human cornea. *Cornea* 1985; 4(3): 157.
26. Dua HS and Shidham VB. Application of specific red blood cell adherence test to the human cornea and conjunctiva. *Am J Ophthalmol* 1979; 88(6): 1067.
27. Ardjomand N, Reich ME and Radner H. Expression of blood group antigens A and/or B in diseased corneas. *Curr Eye Res* 1998; 17(6): 650.
28. Allansmith MR *et al.* ABO Blood groups and corneal transplantation. *Am J Ophthalmol* 1975; 79(3): 493.
29. Roy R *et al.* Role of ABO and Lewis blood group antigens in donor–recipient compatibility of corneal transplantation rejection. *Ophthalmology* 1997; 104(3): 508.

6

The Alloresponse to Corneal Graft

Introduction

Corneal allografts are the most common form of transplantation [1, 2] and enjoy a reputation for high acceptance across major histocompatibility barriers [1, 3, 4] compared to other types of graft. This is based on comparative studies of rejection rates of unmatched corneal grafts versus acute rejection rates of other solid organ, matched transplants. However, acute rejection of grafts such as skin grafts when placed in a previously naïve host follows what is described as a first set rejection response and depending on the MHC, minor-MHC and non-MHC antigen mismatch follows a predictable course of events with rejection usually occurring within the first one to two weeks of graft emplacement. Human corneal grafts do not experience this acute rejection response and thus the first year survival figure of corneal grafts are considerably better [2].

However, corneal graft rejection does occur and when it occurs takes a less rapid course both in humans and experimental models. The five-year survival for human corneal grafts is around 70% [2] compared to 75% or greater for renal allografts [5], showing that long term survival for corneal transplants is actually less than for some solid organ grafts [6]. In both cases, five-year survival figures are a measure of "chronic rejection", a process linked to the indirect mode of allorecognition, unlike acute rejection which is considered to be a consequence of direct allorecognition (see below). Indeed the remarkable improvements in one-year survival of some solid organ grafts has been attributed to the control of acute graft rejection but the long term failure of such grafts due to chronic rejection remains a major obstacle to the overall acceptance rates [7]. However, the definition of chronic rejection is inexact particularly in the clinical evaluation of the distinction between graft failure and chronic graft rejection [8].

Thus it is not surprising that the five-year success rate of corneal allografts is at its present level of around 70%, since corneal grafts are more liable to chronic rejection by the indirect mode and this form of rejection has not been solved for any type of graft. In fact the ten-year survival figures for corneal grafts are even lower (60%) and in their excellent review, Thiel *et al.* point out that up to 50% of corneal grafts undergo rejection at some time [9]. This must be viewed in the context that most corneal grafts are unmatched, that topical steroid immunosuppression is routinely applied in the first weeks to months postgraft and that graft recipient beds differ greatly from high risk to low risk. Thus comparisons of outcome data with other forms of solid organ grafts have to be cautiously interpreted.

Target Antigens in Graft Rejection—Alloantigens and Non-MHC Antigens

Allografts are foreign tissues containing many antigens. The organism responds to foreign antigens by marshalling its immune defences of which there are two broad groups: a rapid reaction force comprising the innate immune response and a more delayed but closely linked adaptive immune response. The innate immune response is generally non-antigen-specific but involves distinct cell types and molecules, and is mediated via particular receptor ligand interactions such as those between Toll receptors and micro-organismal products particularly lipopolysaccharide [10, 11]. The innate immune response has considerable influence on the adaptive immune response and is particularly important in the allograft response (see below).

The adaptive immune response is antigen-specific and can be exquisitely so for specific antigens such as bacterial toxins and viral products. However, alloantigens induce a broader response since they represent species specific polymorphisms, best exemplified by the major histocompatibility (MHC) antigens [11]. MHC antigens were in fact identified through studies of graft rejection in mice and of carefully performed serological studies on human pregnancy sera and are of three broad classes: MHC Class I antigens are present on most nucleated cells but expressed at very different levels and sometimes not at all in the resting state; MHC Class II antigens are typically expressed on professional antigen presenting cells (APC) such as macrophages, B cells and at their highest levels on mature dendritic cells; MHC Class III antigens are represented by complement and heat shock proteins (see Chapter 5). In addition there are minor MHC antigens typified by the H-Y male antigen and non-MHC antigens such as tissue specific antigens which under the appropriate circumstances can behave like autoantigens in transplanted tissues. The numbers of MHC and non-MHC genes and their alleles are constantly being revised and extensive information is available both in review articles and online through the web [11, 12].

The Cellular Response to Allografts—Direct vs Indirect Response

During thymic development most autoreactive T cells are eliminated and the T cell repertoire is shaped to deal with the countless foreign antigens the immune system is likely to meet through the lifetime of the organism. The precursor frequency of such T cells is extremely low but the potential for clonal expansion on antigen encounter is correspondingly high. In addition, some autoreactive T cells avoid clonal deletion in the thymus and escape to the periphery but their precursor frequency is also extremely low and under regulation by peripheral tolerance mechanisms [13]. However, many T cells that primarily react with foreign antigens cross-react with autoantigens thus increasing the risk of autoimmune disease. Since MHC antigens are distributed so widely, presumably to provide generalized tissue-protective immune responses, there is an increased chance of higher frequencies of cross-reactivity with normal T cells as a consequence of allotransplantation. Thus, as many as 2% of the host's T cells have the potential to respond to alloantigens [14] and the alloimmune response to solid organ grafts can be quite marked. In part, the high allorestricted T cell precursor frequency might also be due to the extent of polymorphisms and thus the number of potential "foreign/cross-reactive" antigens present in an allograft. This is reflected in the allospecificity of each graft. MHC Class I and II antigens are considered to be the most potent alloantigens while complement proteins, amongst other mechanisms are important in xenografts [15].

Antigens are recognized by presentation on antigen-presenting cells (APCs), specifically as self MHC-peptide complexes and this applies also to alloantigens. For many foreign antigens this involves presentation of exogenous processed peptide on MHC Class II complexes or shunting of exogenous peptide through the MHC Class I pathway, classically reserved for endogenous peptide (cross presentation) [16]. However, in the case of MHC alloantigen, the MHC Class I and II antigens, usually containing bound self antigens, represent MHC-peptide complexes which do not require processing and are available for presentation directly to CD4+ and CD8+ allospecific T cells. Thus donor cells of the graft themselves can act directly to present alloantigen to host T cells without involving host APCs [17]. This is termed direct presentation of alloantigen and is dependent on the presence of cells within the graft expressing sufficiently high levels of MHC Class I and II [18]. MHC Class I expressing tissue cells can thus activate circulating host CD8+ T cells directly. In addition, direct activation of CD4+ T cells has been ascribed by Lechler to "passenger" leukocytes within the donor graft and there is considerable experimental evidence to support this mechanism particularly in vascularized grafts and in grafts in which there is a high content of resident APCs [7]. In this context, persistence of the direct alloimmune response is clearly dependent on continued expression of MHC Class I antigens by the graft for CD8+ T cells or on survival of donor leukocytes for MHC Class II–CD4+ T cell interactions and MHC Class I–CD8+ T cell cross presentation [19]. Indeed a state of michrochimerism may develop if tissues containing APC stem cell precursors are transplanted, as may occur with bone marrow and liver allografts and paradoxically this is more likely to be associated with transplant tolerance [20].

Until recently, direct allorecognition in corneal allografts, at least through MHC Class II mechanisms, was considered not possible since the central transplanted cornea is devoid of MHC Class II-expressing APCs [21] and even the level of MHC Class I expression is considered to be very low [22]. However, as indicated above, corneal graft rejection both clinically and experimentally does occur and is at least MHC Class I restricted in part [23]. This may be due to cross-presentation of MHC Class I allopeptides from endocytosed donor leukocytes on host APC's to allospecific T cells in the draining lymph node [12, 24]. In contrast the role of donor MHC Class II is much less clear.

Much of the evidence for direct allorecognition has come from *in vitro* studies of the mixed leukocyte response (MLR) (see Chapter 5). *In vivo* evidence for this mechanism of allorejection derives from studies of immunodeficient mice such as SCID or Rag –/– mice, which were also MHC Class I and II negative, reconstituted with syngeneic CD4+ T cells [25]. These mice rejected allogeneic cardiac allografts and, since they contained no CD8+ T cells, this experiment not only demonstrated direct allorecognition *in vivo* but also indicated a requirement for host CD4+ T cells in direct allorecognition rather than CD8+ T cells. This also supports a role for the importance of cross-presentation of alloantigen on APC rather than direct CD8+ T cell recognition of MHC Class I on donor parenchymal cells.

Minor MHC [26] and non-MHC antigens/autoantigens [27, 28] are also important restriction elements in graft rejection and such donor antigen presentation is considered to occur via the indirect route, i.e. the antigens are taken up by host APCs and presented on host MHC Class I and II. MHC alloantigens can also be processed in this way and presented on host APCs as allopeptides; it has been estimated that the frequency of allospecific T cell responses generated via the indirect route is 100-fold lower than via the direct route [23, 29]. In fact this "indirect" mode of antigen presentation is the conventional mechanism for foreign antigen presentation generally.

Indirect alloantigen presentation occurs in all forms of allograft; its recognition has been overshadowed by the rapid and strong direct alloresponse [23] and its importance is only being appreciated as the direct response has become more amenable to control with various immunosuppressive regimes. Indirect allorecognition was initially identified using donor dendritic cell (DC)-depleted kidney allografts in which graft rejection occurred albeit at a slower rate and thus it was suggested that the indirect route might be more relevant for chronic rejection [18]. Indirect allorecognition requires the full participation of the afferent and efferent immune response and thus intact lymphatic communications. Historically, in the cornea these pathways have been thought to be deficient. However, recent studies have shown that mechanisms for indirect allorecognition in the cornea are in place [30].

Thus, although as Streilein puts it, "in corneal allograft rejection the immunogenetic rules do not apply", indicating that the indirect pathway is the predominant pathway for rejection of corneal allografts, the direct pathway also plays some role since depletion of corneal "Langerhans" cells promotes graft acceptance in mice [31], and recent studies have shown that the cornea is rich with passenger leukocytes, which while remaining predominantly MHC Class II negative *in situ*, appear to acquire MHC Class II antigen when they leave the donor cornea and migrate to the draining lymph node after transplantation [32]. In addition, although there is debate over the issue of whether or not tissue matching for MHC Class II antigen permits improved corneal graft acceptance rates [33, 34] (see Chapter 5), a large retrospective study of human corneal graft rejection concluded that donor MHC Class II matching afforded some protection against reversible rejection episodes, indicating a small but significant effect of donor MHC Class II on graft rejection [35] (see also further discussion on this point in Chapter 5).

Mechanism of Graft Rejection

It is self-evident that surgically transplanting tissue from one site to another involves some level of tissue trauma, which will thus induce an inflammatory response. This applies to autologous, syngeneic, allogeneic and xenogeneic grafts and the degree of inflammation varies with the level of trauma (surgical expertise), the size of the graft, the site of the graft, the host response and the level of concomitant micro-organismal contamination during the early healing stage. The overall host response to this variable insult is termed the innate immune response and is characterized by the recruitment and activation of cells of the innate immune system, predominantly myeloid cells and resident tissue bone-marrow derived cells. As indicated above, these cells do not respond to foreign antigens in a specific manner but have sets of receptors which respond to classes of molecules predominantly derived from micro-organisms. These ligands are termed "pathogen-associated molecular patterns" (PAMPs) and their receptors are known as Toll-like receptors (TLRs), following the discovery of their general homology to similar receptors in Drosophila melanogaster [10, 36]. Recent evidence suggests that they may be involved to some extent in the innate immune response to grafts especially xenografts [10, 36].

The innate immune response does not occur in isolation from the adaptive immune response. In fact it has been shown that specific immunity requires innate immune cells (antigen-presenting cells, APCs) to be activated in such a way that they undergo "maturation" before they can induce an adaptive immune response and coexposure to bacterial products such as DNA (CpG motifs), lipoteichoic acid and endotoxin during antigen uptake can promote the adaptive immune response. Thus the greater the innate immune response, the stronger the adaptive immune response. This is particularly relevant to corneal graft rejection where it is known that the skill and experience of the surgeon has a bearing on graft success (see Chapters 2 and 3) and that minor events such as suture removal, development of synechiae or intercurrent infection can initiate the process of graft rejection. This aspect of the effect of surgical trauma on corneal graft rejection has been experimentally addressed and verified for both anterior synechiae and type of sutures [37, 38]. The type of adaptive response may also be determined by the innate immune response. For instance, if corneal graft rejection occurs predominantly via the indirect pathway, there is the potential for immune rejection via three adaptive immune mechanisms: a DTH response (CD4+ T-cell–mediated) within the graft itself, through B cell production of antibody via T cell help in combination with complement, and via induction of cytotoxic CD8+ T cells. In addition, the innate immune response has a considerable role to play by determining the level and type of the T cell response.

The afferent immune response to corneal allografts

The afferent arm of the immune response to corneal allograft comprises several stages, including induction of the innate immune response, antigen transport from the cornea to the secondary lymphoid tissue, processing and presentation of antigen by antigen-presenting cells (APCs) and transmission of the message to T cells.

The innate immune response

Corneal graft rejection is a cell-mediated process, involving T cells, i.e. the process involves the adaptive immune response. There may be an added humoral component in "high risk" situations [39, 40] but this is usually small and is not essential, since graft rejection can occur in B-cell and complement-deficient mice [41]. As indicated above, this adaptive immune T cell response is initiated by an earlier innate immune response of the host to the presence of the allograft but the nature of the innate immune response has not been studied in great detail.

In human corneal grafts, there are obvious reasons for a lack of information concerning the cellular infiltration during either the innate response or even the acute phase of the adaptive graft rejection response since sampling of tissue for histological analysis is ethically difficult. However, there has been one study of the cellular content of the aqueous humour during acute graft rejection episodes. In this study monocytes and lymphocytes were identified in increasing numbers with severity of the rejection episode but granulocytes were infrequent [42]. These data suggest that rejection episodes in human corneal graft correlate with the adaptive immune response.

Several studies of irreversibly rejected human corneal grafts have been performed usually after a prolonged period of clinical rejection and these reveal a mixed infiltration of cells belonging to both the innate and the adaptive immune responses, including dendritic cells (Figure 6.1) [43]. In addition, considerable apoptosis of keratocytes has been observed indicating possible effector mechanisms in this situation [44]. However, mechanistic analysis of this data is limited.

Most information concerning the cellular infiltrate of the graft has come from studies of experimental corneal graft in a variety of species including sheep, rabbit, guinea pig, rat and mouse (see Chapter 8). However, there have been surprisingly few studies of the earliest response of the host to experimental corneal allografts at a time when it might be expected that the innate immune response could be studied in isolation, prior to the onset of the adaptive response. Until recently, most studies examined the cellular infiltrate of the tissues around the time of clinical rejection [45–54] or occasionally at an earlier time in the developing immune response for instance at 1–2 days postgrafting [45]. Presumably it was considered that nothing much happened until there was a detectable adaptive immune response.

However, there is from the beginning of graft emplacement a significant innate immune response [30]. Cells of the innate immune system include

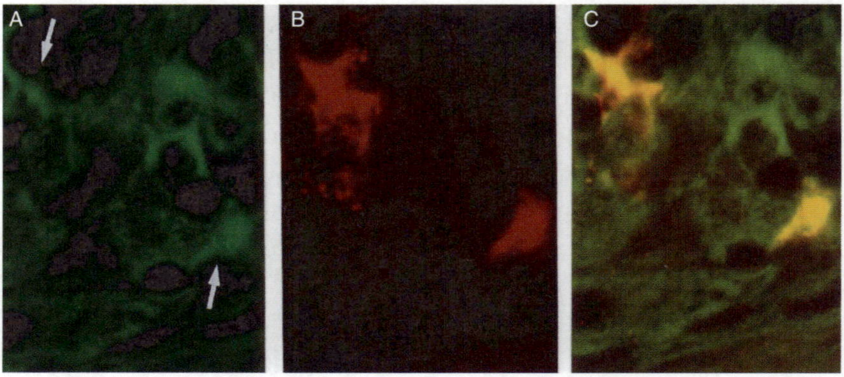

Figure 6.1 CD1a/MHC class II positive dendritic cells in the stroma of the rejected human corneal graft. (**A**) MHC class II (FITC staining); (**B**) CD1a (Texas red staining); (**C**) merged image.

neutrophils, macrophages, dendritic cells and other cells such as NK and NKT cells, and tissue mast cells. Within minutes of grafting, there is a significant inflammatory response (Figure 6.2) in the form of neutrophil infiltration. Macrophages are also an early component of the cellular infiltrate both in syngeneic and in allogeneic grafts [30]. In addition, they have an important role in rejection overall since depletion of macrophages leads to prolonged acceptance of grafts in both quiet eyes and in "high risk" grafts [55, 56]. In allogeneic grafts their role as both effectors and inducers has recently been highlighted (Slegers, personal communication).

Bone-marrow-derived dendritic cells (DCs) are also an important early entrant into the inflammatory cell infiltrate although their numbers are low. Their role in antigen presentation is central to the adaptive immune response (see below).

NK cells and NKT cells arrive after 1–3 days and their role in graft rejection is acquiring increasing relevance. NK cells (CD3–, CD8+, TCR–, CD16+) are designed to kill virus-infected cells and tumour cells which they do by one of two broad mechanisms: Fas/TNF : FasL/TNFr

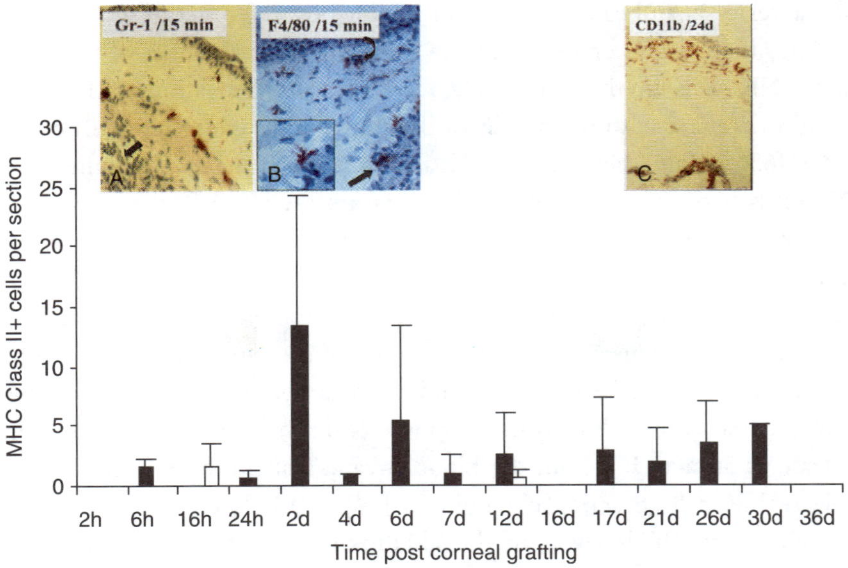

Figure 6.2 Immunohistochemical quantitative analysis of MHC class II positive cells infiltrating mouse corneal graft during rejection process. (**Inset A**) Gr-1 positive neutrophils at 15 minutes post-corneal-transplantation; (**inset B**) F4/80 positive macrophages at 15 minutes post-corneal-transplantation; (**inset C**) CD11b positive macrophages at 24 days post-corneal-transplantation. (Filled bars—allogeneic grafts; empty bars—syngeneic grafts.)

mechanisms or perforin-mediated granule exocytosis [57]. The role of NK cells in solid organ graft rejection has recently been highlighted in a model of cardiac transplantation [58]. Only by blockade of both innate NK cells and adaptive CD28+ T cells could long term survival of the grafts be achieved, thus highlighting both the importance of NK cells in the overall immune response to allografts but also the inextricable linkage of the innate and the adaptive immune systems. Interestingly, although both systems are involved in graft rejection, activation of the innate immune system alone is sufficient to induce graft rejection [59].

The role of NK cells in corneal graft rejection is relatively unexplored. Previous studies have shown that NK cells are absent from the normal (donor) cornea [60] but occur in experimental corneal grafts in the early phase after grafting [45]. NK cells are inhibited by MHC Class I antigens through the KIR (human) and Ly49 receptors (mouse) [57] and the low or absent levels of MHC Class I in the cornea render this tissue liable to attack by activated NK cells. However, recent studies have shown that the anterior chamber of the eye contains an anti-NK cell property mediated by a molecule which is similar if not identical to macrophage migration inhibitory factor [61, 62]. TGFβ which is also present in high amounts in the anterior chamber of the eye can inhibit NK cell function (see below).

Thus there are several mechanisms in the anterior chamber of the eye to keep NK cells in their normally inactive state. Activation of NK cells requires contact with other cells of the innate immune system particularly DCs [63] before they can participate in tissue damage. In homeostasis, NK cells have the potential to kill immature DCs due to their low levels of surface MHC Class I but after maturation, surface-expressing MHC Class I+ DCs not only are resistant to NK cell attack but reciprocally activate NK cells via specific receptors. In this way the interaction between NK cells and DCs is central to the amplification of the innate immune response and provides a link between this and the adaptive immune response [64]. An essential component to this response is tissue damage and chemokine release to attract DCs from the blood stream. Immature DCs (iDCs) then release NK cell attracting chemokines [64] (see below). Finally, NK cells which express high levels of the chemokine receptor CCR7 have the potential to migrate to the draining lymph node where they can exert "quality control" over mature DC which may express less than optimal levels of MHC Class I [64].

Thus several cell types enter the cornea during the early innate immune response to allograft: neutrophils, macrophages, NK cells and DCs. The route of entry of cells to the different layers of the cornea is of some interest since the endothelium is the major determinant of corneal clarity and is therefore the most critical target tissue. Cells entering the stroma and the epithelium appear to migrate from vessels close to the limbus. It has been shown that resident limbal Langerhans cells migrate into the central cornea during the first few hours after grafting [31, 65–72]. However, the marked increase in myeloid cells including DCs, in corneal grafts in the early stages after grafting is likely to be induced by recent emigrants from the bone marrow.

In contrast to the stroma and epithelium, cells contacting the endothelium appear to traverse the anterior chamber from the iris using the fibrin clot that develops at this site from 24 hours after grafting. Previous studies have in fact shown that there is a very large increase in the numbers of iris macrophages and MHC Class II positive cells in the iris in the first hours after corneal allografting [46, 49], thus providing a source of innate immune cells, and macrophages are conspicuous on the endothelium from an early stage (Figure 6.3). It is likely therefore that they traverse the anterior chamber

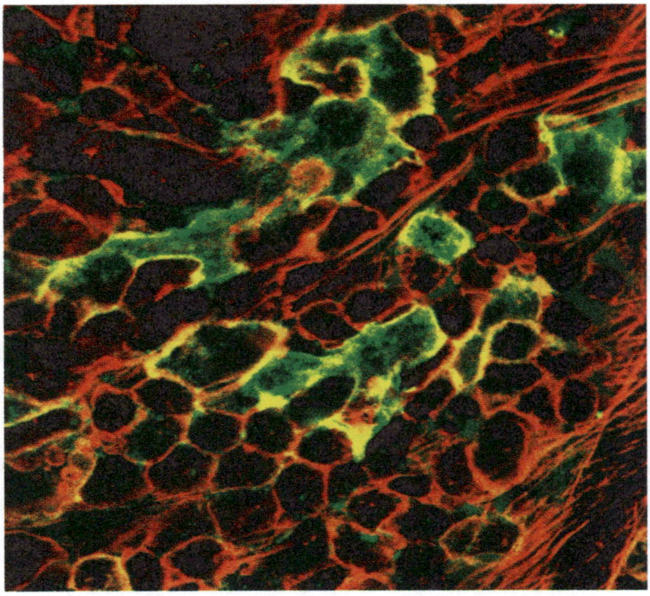

Figure 6.3 Corneal endothelial cell monolayer from a mouse donor corneal graft six days post-corneal-transplantation, showing normal hexagonal shaped endothelial cells and abnormal cell forms stained with PI (red) labelled anti-intracellular actin mAb and FITC labelled anti-F4/80 (green) mAb staining for macrophages.

from the uveal tract directly onto the endothelium through the matrix of the fibrin clot. Macrophages continue to increase in numbers in allogeneic grafts compared to syngeneic grafts and are likely to be important as effectors of endothelial cell damage (see below). Fibrin clots on failed human corneal grafts have been recognised for many years and this mechanism for access of cells to the corneal endothelium would seem to be a general one amongst species [53].

Macrophages have traditionally been regarded as secondary antigen presenting cells, DCs being most relevant in the induction of naïve T cells. However, recent studies have shown that depletion of macrophages, particularly at the earliest stages after graft emplacement, prevents graft rejection (see above) indicating that macrophages may also have a role at this stage.

Antigen transport from the cornea

Induction of the adaptive immune response requires (allo)antigen to be transported to the secondary lymphoid tissue for presentation to naïve, antigen specific T cells. Until recently, it was considered that the eye (and the brain) did not have a lymphatic supply and that contact with the secondary lymphoid tissue occurred through the spleen [73]. In addition, antigen transported to the spleen was considered to induce tolerance (ACAID; see below) rather than immunity and this remains one of the central facets of ocular immune privilege (see below) [73]. However, recent studies have shown that antigen inoculated into the eye drains to the submandibular lymph node [74] and this lymph node appears to be essential for priming the immune response to corneal alloantigen. In addition, within two hours of graft emplacement there is a dramatic fall in the percentage of activated CD4+ and CD8+ T cells in the draining submandibular lymph node [30]. Draining lymph node (DLN) T cells then go through repeated but diminishing cycles of expansion and contraction which peter out at a time coincident with clinical signs of graft rejection [30]. At the same time, there is an increase in the numbers of antigen presenting DCs and macrophages trafficking to the (DLN) which upregulate their complement of costimulatory molecules [30].

These data strongly point towards an early and rapid transport of alloantigen to the DLN after corneal graft emplacement which is then presented to allospecific T cells. The repeated cycles of T cell clonal expansion and emigration from the lymph node have been interpreted as reflecting the generation of a sufficient frequency of activated effector T cells trafficking to the cornea to cause such damage to the corneal endothelium that immunological rejection becomes clinically apparent [30].

Further experiments have confirmed that antigen is indeed rapidly transported to the draining lymph node within antigen presenting cells. Using a model of corneal graft in immunodeficient mice reconstituted with T cells specific for the murine C5 peptide, it has been shown that application to the donor cornea of a plasmid containing the C5 peptide sequence, tagged with a GFP label, led to the specific expression of GFP label in CD11c positive DCs in the draining submandibular node within 6h of grafting. In addition there was an early activation of C5 specific T cells in the DLN. In contrast, GFP label did not appear in the spleen until 24–48 hours after grafting (Kuffová *et al.*, in preparation).

How do antigen-presenting cells traffic from the eye to the draining lymph node? Although lymphatic vessels coursing from the eye are difficult to identify, functional studies suggest that there is a lymphatic communication via the uveoscleral drainage pathway from the intraocular compartment [75] and special staining using an antibody to VEGFcr have shown that lymphangiogenesis can occur rapidly particularly after corneal grafting in "high risk" situations. Furthermore anti-VEGF antibodies inhibit graft rejection and may do so by delaying development of new lymphatics [76].

The antigen-presenting cell—accessory molecules CD40 and costimulation

Presentation of antigen for induction of the adaptive immune response might occur *in situ* within the tissues or after transport of antigen to the draining lymph node. Antigen presentation on MHC Class I to cytotoxic CD8+ T cells by tissue resident corneal cells, such as keratocytes [77] and endothelial cells, is a likely mechanism for cytotoxic T cell damage to these cells but requires upregulation of MHC Class I by these cells. However, since CD4+ T cells are necessary for corneal graft rejection by the indirect alloimmune response [78–80], professional APCs utilizing MHC Class II are required and, at least for the initiation of the disease, this takes place in the DLN.

The increase in DCs in the DLN soon after corneal grafting almost certainly reflects the increased in recruitment of myeloid cells to the cornea from the bone marrow, itself induced by the inflammatory stimulus (see above innate immune response). Myeloid cell recruitment to the cornea also goes through a cyclical pattern, almost in phase shift with the activated T cell population changes in the DLN [30]. APCs also upregulate their markers for CD40 and B7 and it is likely that this is in part induced by T cell CD40L and CD28/CTLA4 [27, 81–83]. A number of studies have shown that CD40:CD40L interactions modify the strength of the corneal allograft response but are not essential for graft rejection since rejection occurs, albeit delayed, in CD40 KO mice [84] (Kuffová *et al.*, in preparation). Several other inhibitory and co-stimulatory accessory molecule ligand-receptor pairs such as ICOS, OX40 and PD-1 (and their ligands) [85, 86] are likely to be involved in the overall alloimmune response and will play a part in the eventual outcome. In particular, the role of the CD28/CTLA4:B7.1 B7.2 complex is interesting. CD28 is constitutively expressed by T cells and is important in the initial priming response to antigen [85]. In contrast, CTLA4 is normally at low levels in resting T cells and is upregulated during the first 48 hours after APC–T cell contact. Signalling through the CTLA4 molecule generally downregulates the T cell response and is important in terminating the immune response. Recent work in tumour cell biology and immunotherapy for metastatic tumours has shown that blockade CTLA-4 by specific antibody therapy permits DC vaccination mediated induction of antitumour immunity [87–89].

In a similar way, it is self-evident that the final outcome of the T cell response to alloantigen and to antigens generally is fine-tuned in several aspects.

Transmitting the message to T cells

Transmission of the message by APCs to T cells in the DLN requires APC to migrate to the T cell area of the DLN and to interact there with their cognate ligand. As indicated above, T cells are activated within two hours of corneal grafting and by 24 hours have undergone considerable expansion. Studies of APC–T cell interactions indicate that several "hits" are required before full activation of the T cell [90, 91] and this would fit with the kinetics of the response seen in the corneal allograft response. However, the repeated cycles of T cell activation and emigration indicate that there must be a constant supply of antigen-loaded APCs migrating to the DLN where they activate successive rounds of naïve T cells recirculating from the blood stream (Figure 6.4). Thus the persistence of the allograft and the constant source of alloantigen presented by trafficking APCs are part of the reason for strength of the alloimmune response.

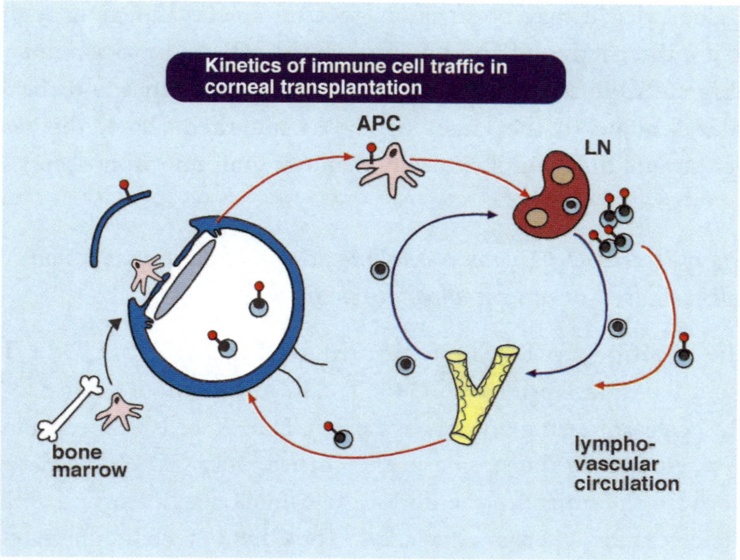

Figure 6.4 Diagram of the kinetics of immune cell traffic in corneal transplantation. Placement of donor corneal graft into the recipient host bed induces migration of antigen-presenting cells (APCs) from the bone marrow to the graft where they pick up antigen and transport it to the draining lymph nodes (LN). This leads to activation of allospecific T cells, which normally recirculate through the blood-lymph circulation, but after activation home to the target tissue, namely to the donor graft (red dots with bar represent alloantigen).

The efferent immune response

The efferent arm of the immune response also involves a series of steps, including expansion and emigration of T cells from the DLN, homing of T cells to the graft, differential function of subsets of T cells (CD4 vs CD8), cytokine release and effector macrophage programming, and finally tissue damage.

Expansion and emigration of T cells from the DLN

The rapid fall in activated CD8+ and CD4+ T cells that occurs after grafting [30] may reflect the high numbers of alloreactive T cells present in the organism (see above). In addition, although the indirect pathway is considered to be mainly operating in the corneal allograft response, the recent evidence that MHC Class II-donor leukocytes, which are normally present in the cornea, migrate to the DLN and there express donor MHC Class II, opens the possibility that some level of direct allopresentation may also occur, albeit that it may be small and not sustained [32]. Antigen-specific T cells are then activated and undergo clonal expansion to a point where they migrate from the DLN into the efferent lymphatics and the blood stream and home to the target organ. As indicated above, this cycle is repeated several times until clinically manifest graft rejection occurs [30].

Homing of T cells to the graft—cytokines, chemokines and adhesion molecules involved in corneal allograft rejection

In the target organ, T cells are first detected by day 2–3, CD8+ T cells arriving a few hours prior to CD4+ T cells in one mouse study [30] but CD8+ T cells appearing several days after CD4+ T cells in sheep allografts [92]. Interestingly in the stroma of the cornea, only CD4+ T cells appear to cross from the host into the donor graft in allogeneic corneas unlike in syngeneic corneas when neither CD4+ or CD8+ T cells appear to infiltrate the donor [30].

How are T cells induced to migrate towards the target tissue? In vascularised grafts it has recently been shown that there is a marked macrophage infiltration and increase in cytokines and chemokines within 24 hours of grafting as part of the innate immune response and this provides the link with the adaptive immune response [59]. In the rat cornea [93], there is an early upregulation of several cytokines and chemokines including IL-1β, IL-6, IL-10, IL-12 p40, and MIP-2 with little difference between syngeneic and allogeneic responses. Thus this probably represents a typical injury response and is reflected in the myeloid cell infiltration seen in both types of grafts [30]. In syngeneic grafts, levels of cytokines decreased after about 6–9 days but in allografts they continued to rise particularly TGF-β1, TGF-β2, and IL-1RA. IL-4, IL-13, and IFN-γ were detected only during the phase of clinical rejection suggesting that populations of these cells had reached a level at which cytokine production was detectable. In other studies in the mouse, MIP-1β and RANTES have been shown to be important in corneal allograft rejection. In addition, TNF-α appears to be important for the migration of Langerhans cells to the centre of the cornea [66]. Similar studies in the sheep indicate that there is an upregulation of IFN-γ and TNF-α in allografts but not in autografts [92].

Although no specific studies have been performed as yet in corneal allograft rejection, information from other systems in transplantation, and immune mediated disease generally, indicate that specific chemokines are likely to attract distinct populations of cells not only to the target organ but also in the essential trafficking of APCs and T cells between the tissue and the secondary lymphoid organs. Thus DCs express CCR1, CCR5 and CCR6 in the immature state and are attracted to sites of inflammation via release of cytokines such as MIP-1α, MIP-1β, MIP-3α and IP-10; as they mature, DCs upregulate CCR7 when migrating to the DLN where they bind to their cognate ligand SLC [94, 95]. After DC contact with T cells and T cell activation, effector T cells downregulate their expression of L selectin allowing them to emigrate from the DLN and home to the tissue.

There is also a co-ordinated and regulated expression of adhesion molecules and their respective ligands by both cells of the tissue and trafficking leukocytes during allograft rejection. Thus ICAM-1 and 3:LFA-1 and VCAM:VLA4 interactions appear to be important mediators of corneal allograft rejection since monoclonal antibody blockade of either or both ligand-receptor pairs prolongs allograft survival [96] and is associated with reduced Th1 cytokines in the graft and impaired DTH responses [97].

The overall sequence of events in T cell homing to the target tissue thus appears to be an early, if not almost instant, expression of chemokines by parenchymal and invading cells of the tissue, followed rapidly by increased expression of selectins, and later integrins, permitting firm adhesion and migration of the inflammatory cells into the tissue.

Role of CD4+ and CD8+ T cells

Traditionally, CD8+ cytotoxic T cells are considered important mediators of allograft rejection, particularly in the context of the direct alloimmune response. In the cornea, where the indirect alloresponse is predominant, CD4+ T cells appear to be required for allograft rejection while CD8+ T cells are not. Thus, corneal grafts survive indefinitely in CD4KO mice while rejection proceeds normally in CD8 KO mice [98, 99]. Cytotoxic T cell responses can be elicited in mice with corneal allografts particularly when placed heterotopically [100] but the predominance of the CD4+ T cell response was first shown by Joo *et al.* [101] and their critical role in corneal allograft rejection was revealed by Hašková *et al.* [79]. CD8+ T cells appear to have a relatively independent role in rejecting skin grafts but only a minor role in corneal allograft rejection. In particular, recent work in perforin KO mice, presumed to be central to CD8+ T cell cytotoxicity, has shown that corneal graft rejection is not inhibited [102]. The importance of CD4+ T cells is underlined by the observation that

CD4+ T cells enter the allografts but not isografts [30, 103] and in this regard they may be important in recruiting other effector cells.

T cell function in the graft—cytokine release and macrophage programming

T cells and myeloid cells have a reciprocal relationship in the allograft response. On the one hand, myeloid cells are the early infiltrating cells in graft rejection and, either directly or through interaction with parenchymal cells, release (a) chemokines such as IP-10 and MIG which are important in T cell recruitment and (b) cytokines which are inducers of Th1 cell activation such as IL-12, IL-15, IL-18 and 23 [104]. Conversely, T cells release cytokines such as IFN-γ and TNF-α and chemokines which are activators and inducers of macrophages [105]. In addition, other cells such as NK cells, neutrophils and mast cells contribute to the cellular cross talk.

In the face of such bewildering complexity it can be difficult to dissect out specific mechanisms. However, these are not broad spectrum effects. For instance, INF-γ produced either by NK cells or T cells is important in inducing monocytes to release MIG, which in turn has a direct effect on T cell recruitment into cardiac allografts [103, 106]. IP-10 although similarly regulated does not have this effect [103]. In addition, it would appear that allospecific T cells have greater potential to activate macrophages that the T cells which migrate albeit in lower numbers into syngeneic grafts [30].

Cytotoxic T cells add to this overall response, by inducing *in situ* cell death and promoting for instance keratocyte apoptosis [44]. Interestingly, uptake of apoptotic cells by macrophages and DCs is more likely to lead to tolerance than immunity [107] and cell death under these circumstances may have a downregulatory effect on the overall inflammatory response.

Mechanism of tissue damage

Tissue destruction in corneal allograft rejection occurs at a cellular level with each of the three main cellular components contributing to immunogenicity. Studies in the genetically modified GFP mouse have shown that the epithelium is completely replaced within the first week of grafting whether it be a syngeneic or allogeneic graft. This implies a non-adaptive immune response, and in fact may in one sense reflect an accelerated turnover of epithelial cells in response to trauma similar to what might occur after epithelial debridement. A true alloimmune response, however, can be elicited to donor epithelial cells and is in part related to the complement of donor Langerhans cells [108].

The stromal cells (keratocytes and donor leukocytes [32, 60]) are also the subject of immunological attack and undergo apoptosis [44], presumably mediated by infiltrating myeloid and T cells.

The main focus of attack is, however, the endothelium. Studies in the GFP mouse indicate that donor endothelium survives in accepted grafts, even if these corneas have been through a period of transient "rejection" as evidenced by a clinical corneal opacity score greater than two and usually occurring about 10–15 days after grafting [108]. In contrast, in eyes in which there has been persistent corneal opacification without recovery for a prolonged period of time (usually more than eight weeks), there is usually complete loss of the donor endothelium with no evidence of repopulation of the donor from host endothelium [108]. It would thus appear that the endothelium, under attack by immune cells migrating from the iris across the anterior chamber in the interstices of the fibrin clot, undergoes a period of transient dysfunction leading to opacification. However, at this stage the endothelium is not lost and has the power to recover, provided the immunological attack can be checked [37]. Presumably, this occurs by mechanisms such as Fas-FasL interactions (see below) and depends greatly on the level and type of immune cell attack.

There is a wide range of cells which can cause endothelial cell damage including neutrophils, NK cells, macrophages, and T cells. Some of these cause damage directly such as cytotoxic T cells, NK cells and macrophages while others operate indirectly, such as CD4+ T cells, and subsets of NK cells (activating DCs; see above under *innate immunity*). The relative contribution of effector cells in corneal allograft rejection is unclear but, as indicated above, CD8+ T cells are relatively unimportant while macrophage depletion experiments indicate that these cells have a significant role [55, 56]. Certainly, the posterior surface of rejected corneal grafts besides having no endothelium is extensively covered with macrophages (Figure 6.3). If macrophages do have a major role to play, the clinical differentiation between graft failure (due to endothelial cell damage and loss) and immunological graft rejection becomes blurred.

A role for B cells, antibodies and complement in allograft rejection has also been investigated but unlike in xenografts where natural antibodies and complement play a major role (see Chapter 7), there seems to be little part to play by these mechanisms in corneal allograft rejection under normal circumstances [41]. However, antibody and complement mediated mechanisms are not disabled and donor corneal damage via this route is possible [39].

Ocular Immune Privilege

Introduction

Immune privilege is a term applied to sites or tissue in which the full immunodestructive response is modified. The term was first applied to the eye by Medawar and colleagues (for review see [109]), who found that allogeneic transplants placed in the anterior chamber of the eye survived considerably longer that similar skin allografts. Further studies by Streilein, Kaplan and Niederkorn confirmed the immunologically privileged status of the anterior chamber of the eye by showing that certain allogeneic tumours when placed in the skin were rapidly rejected but when placed in the anterior chamber not only survived but proliferated and metastasized [110, 111].

Streilein and Kaplan further showed that inoculation of antigen into the anterior chamber of the eye led to a deviated immune response in that rechallenge with the same antigen systemically was associated with a reduced delayed type hypersensitivity (DTH) response, although certain antibody responses and cytotoxic T cell responses to rechallenge remained intact [112]. They described this form of tolerance induction as Anterior Chamber Associated Immune Deviation (ACAID) and similar altered immune responses to rechallenge have been described for other tissues such as the testis [113], the brain [114] and the pancreas [115, 116]. In contrast, rechallenge after primary inoculation of antigen in the skin with adiuvant usually induces a memory response (shorter interval and stronger response; see below). Primary inoculation of antigen into skin (subcutaneous injection) without adiuvant or intravenously is frequently associated with antigen specific tolerance but it is believed that the ACAID response has features which set it apart. In addition, it has been suggested that the ACAID response to eye-inoculated antigen is a paradigm for nonresponsiveness to endogenous "sequestered" antigens such as retinal autoantigens [116].

Immune privilege and the cornea

Several mechanisms have been invoked to account for ocular immune privilege. These include the blood-ocular barrier and in particular, for the retina, the blood-retinal barrier since this is similar in many ways to the blood-brain barrier. However, most functional studies of these barriers have been performed in relation to the passive passage of molecules of different sizes, and cells traverse vascular barriers by active means. Since both retinal and brain inflammation occur clinically and experimentally, these barriers would seem to be relatively easily breached by inflammatory cells.

Suggested defects in the afferent arm of the immune response for instance through lack of lymphatic channels (see above) or lack of resident ocular APCs [117–122] have been disproved. The retina proper appears not to contain DCs but does contain immunoregulatory cells in the form of microglia [123]. The cornea also has been shown to contain many CD45+ and CD11c+ cells which appear to express MHC Class II when they traffic to the DLN [32] (see above).

The most likely explanations therefore for the immunologically privileged status of the intact eye relate to aspects of the tissue itself and the surrounding milieu. Several studies have shown that apoptosis-inducing mechanisms involving constitutive expression of molecules such as FasL and TRAIL operate in promoting cell death in invading Fas and TRAIL-L+ cells, such as lymphocytes, into the anterior chamber [124–126]. In addition, the anterior chamber contains high concentrations of molecules such as TGF-β and a range of neuropeptides such as α-MSH, VIP, CGRP, free endogenous cortisol and other molecules which are known to have immunomodulatory roles (for review see [73]). Thus cells which enter the eye are at risk of cell death or at least of entering a state of anergy, promoted by one or all of these mechanisms. Some of these systems have a dual role and can in fact promote inflammation such as Fas-FasL [127]. For instance it has been shown that rejection of tumours in the eye depends critically on whether the tumour expresses soluble or membrane bound FasL [127]. The role of Fas in immune privileged sites can thus be amphipathic [128].

Immune privilege and corneal graft

The prolonged acceptance of fully mismatched experimental corneal allografts compared to skin grafts and similar results in the first year survival of unmatched human corneal grafts has been attributed to ocular immune privilege, and ACAID itself has been proposed as a mechanism. Initally this was correlated with the avascularity of the cornea and the lack of passenger leukocytes. In the case of the former explanation, there is considerable evidence to show that placing a clear corneal graft into a "high risk" vascularized host bed reduces significantly the chances of acceptance [1, 2].

However, in this situation it is clearly not donor vessels and their MHC antigens which are the target of attack, as they are for other vascularized organs involving direct allorecognition [18], and thus the explanation for reduced graft survival in this situation must relate to aspects of the host efferent response. The recent evidence that donor corneas do contain a population of passenger leukocytes [32] suggests that some degree of direct allorecognition may occur but indirect allorecogntion in corneal graft rejection is predominant (see above).

This of itself may be sufficient to explain the prolonged survival of corneal allografts. Indirect allorecognition is considered to be the basis of chronic rejection which occurs in most types of allografts provided the acute rejection response can be controlled (see above). Therefore, if there is no or only a minimal direct alloresponse to the cornea, a chronic delayed response to corneal allografts would be expected. In fact the five-year survival (chronic rejection) of corneal grafts compared to renal grafts is remarkably similar and does not suggest a privileged status for the cornea from chronic rejection. The lack of acute rejection in the cornea (i.e. rejection occurring in a naïve host within two weeks as occurs in skin allografts) can thus be simply attributed to the lack of significant expression of MHC antigens.

The indirect alloresponse to corneal grafts is, however, likely to be modified. Firstly, the overall antigen load is low. Secondly, the lack of blood vessels helps to prevent the efferent immune response despite the positive sensitizing afferent response. Thirdly, the immunosuppressive milieu of the anterior chamber of the eye (see above [73]), although likely to be disrupted during the first weeks after grafting, has the potential to re-establish itself and may thus play a later role provided the initial trauma and the accompanying innate immune response is minimized. Thus the immunosuppressive microenvironment of the anterior chamber of the eye is likely to modulate the already less pronounced indirect alloimmune response.

A role for ACAID in modulating indirect allorecognition to a graft placed in a naïve host is more difficult to accommodate into this process. ACAID is antigen specific and requires prior sensitisation of the host to the donor alloantigens and under such circumstances, can delay graft rejection [129, 130]. Clearly this does not apply to naïve hosts. As Thiel *et al.* nicely phrase it, "The questions of whether a corneal graft can itself induce ACAID without the clinically inapplicable requirement for previous priming of the recipient, and whether induction of ACAID is fast enough to compete with graft-mediated host sensitization, remain unanswered" [9].

Mechanism of tolerance

The eye thus has two mechanisms of downregulating the immune response: (a) it can inhibit activated effector T cells which enter the eye, for example through its apoptosis-inducing mechanisms (see above), and (b) it can tolerize T cells systemically before they reach the eye (ACAID). The mechanism of systemic tolerance mediated through the ocular compartments and tissues has generated much investigation. There is evidence that after antigen inoculation into the eye, antigen-specific tolerizing signals are transported in the blood stream to the spleen via antigen presenting cells which interact in a multicellular cluster involving NKT cells, CD4+ T cells, and B cells to generate CD8+ T suppressor or regulatory cells (see review in [131]). How ocular APCs reach the spleen in sufficient numbers is not clear but there also appears to be some involvement of trafficking to the thymus [132].

Whether similar mechanisms operate in corneal graft rejection is not known. However, it has been established that splenectomy accelerates corneal graft rejection [133], indicating that some central mechanism is involved in the orchestration of the ocular tolerance response.

Memory and Induction of Tolerance

Rechallenge of the host with a second graft is likely to promote more rapid rejection of the graft and clinically this is well recognized by the poor survival of regrafts even after close MHC matching [2, 6]. This is evidence of immunological memory defined as a faster and stronger response to rechallenge with the same antigen [134]. The time interval between the first and the second graft is important in that the longer the interval the less likely the chance of graft rejection but memory is still long-lived and difficult to manage.

Experiments in mice using GFP label and a murine complement (C5) DNA in a Rag –/– model system [135] indicate that corneal-graft-related memory cells reside in the spleen as shown by antigen-specific $CD62L^{lo}CD44^{hi}$ cells more than 30 days after application of the C5 containing donor graft (Kuffová *et al.,* in preparation). Interestingly, the level of alloantigenic disparity and possibly the total antigen load may have an influence on this response. For instance, corneal grafts with single disparity at the H-Y locus fail to induce rejection even if there is subsequent exposure to and rejection of H-Y disparate skin grafts [136]. Despite this, T cell memory induction via skin grafting prevents acceptance of a corneal graft to the second eye even though the original corneal graft is not rejected. Thus memory is effective in inducing graft rejection unless immunological privilege has been re-established [136].

Attempts to promote immunologically tolerance to corneal alloantigens involving prior exposure to donor antigen, e.g. intravenous infusion of donor spleen cells, or oral administration of donor corneal or spleen cells has also been attempted and has shown some success [137–139]. In part this may be due to the induction of T regulatory cells, as has been shown for other mucosally delivered antigens [140], but the precise mechanism remains unclear. In addition, the risk of inducing immunity rather than tolerance exists using these methods [141]. In other systems, use of monoclonal antibodies and other means of inducing infectious tolerance [142] has been through upregulation of T regulatory cells particularly cells of the CD4+CD25+ variety [143]. In addition, attempts to promote tolerance through such means using donor antigen pulsed-DCs has shown some success [144].

At present, studies of these methods in corneal graft are at an early stage. Several methods have been used to prevent or delay experimental graft rejection using monoclonal antibodies but the induction of long term tolerance using such means has not been particularly successful (see Chapter 10).

Conclusion

In summary, the immune response to corneal allografts is initiated by a very early developing innate immune response which is inextricably linked to induction of the adaptive response. In corneal allograft rejection, the indirect mode of alloantigen presentation (including presentation of MHC and minor/non-MHC antigens) by host antigen-presenting cells, particularly DCs, predominates, although there may be a small component of direct allorecognition of MHC antigens. The strength of the adaptive response loosely correlates with the severity of the innate immune response and factors such as surgical trauma, nature of the suture material and associated micro-organismal contamination play a significant part in the outcome of the graft. Even if the initial period of host sensitization is successfully negotiated, late graft rejection can be induced by a nonspecific innate immune insult such as suture abscess (see Chapter 3) or even more remotely by vaccination for unrelated disease such as flu [145].

Corneal grafts do not enjoy as much "privilege" in the classical sense as was previously thought but probably have a good initial success rate even if fully mismatched, due to the fact that direct allorecognition does not play a major part in rejection. In contrast the late rejection rates for cornea are similar to those of other solid organ grafts and represent a mixture of chronic (indirect) graft rejection and functional graft failure.

References

1. The collaborative corneal transplantation studies (CCTS): effectiveness of histocompatibility matching in high-risk corneal transplantation. The Collaborative Corneal Transplantation Studies Research Group. *Arch Ophthalmol* 1992; 110(10): 1392.
2. The Australian Corneal Graft Registry: 1990 to 1992 report. *Aust N Z J Ophthalmol* 1993; 21(2 Suppl): 1.
3. Roelen DL *et al.* The presence of activated donor HLA class I-reactive T lymphocytes is associated with rejection of corneal grafts. *Transplantation* 1995; 59(7): 1039.
4. Hahn AB *et al.* The association of lymphocytotoxic antibodies with corneal allograft rejection in high risk patients. The Collaborative Corneal Transplantation Studies Research Group. *Transplantation* 1995; 59(1): 21.
5. Nicholson ML *et al.* A comparison of the results of renal transplantation from non-heart-beating, conventional cadaveric, and living donors. *Kidney Int* 2000; 58(6): 2585.
6. Williams KA *et al.* How successful is corneal transplantation? A report from the Australian Corneal Graft Register. *Eye* 1995; 9(Pt 2): 219.
7. Game DS, Warrens AN and Lechler RI. Rejection mechanisms in transplantation. *Wien Klin Wochenschr* 2001; 113(20–21): 832.
8. Halloran PF. Call for revolution: a new approach to describing allograft deterioration. *Am J Transplant* 2002; 2(3): 195.
9. Thiel MA, Coster DJ and Williams KA. The potential of antibody-based immunosuppressive agents for corneal transplantation. *Immunol Cell Biol* 2003; 81(2): 93.
10. Gordon S. Pattern recognition receptors: doubling up for the innate immune response. *Cell* 2002; 111(7): 927.
11. Robinson J and Marsh SG. The IMGT/HLA sequence database. *Rev Immunogenet* 2000; 2(4): 518.
12. Simpson E *et al.* Minor H antigens: genes and peptides. *Transpl Immunol* 2002; 10(2–3): 115.
13. Goldschneider I and Cone RE. A central role for peripheral dendritic cells in the induction of acquired thymic tolerance. *Trends Immunol* 2003; 24(2): 77.
14. Breur-Vriesendorp BS *et al.* Frequency analysis of HLA-specific cytotoxic T lymphocyte precursors in humans. *Transplantation* 1991; 51(5): 1096.
15. Garrovillo M, Ali A and Oluwole SF. Indirect allorecognition in acquired thymic tolerance: induction of donor-specific tolerance to rat cardiac allografts by allopeptide-pulsed host dendritic cells. *Transplantation* 1999; 68(12): 1827.

16. Nelson D, Bundell C and Robinson B. In vivo cross-presentation of a soluble protein antigen: kinetics, distribution, and generation of effector CTL recognizing dominant and subdominant epitopes. *J Immunol* 2000; 165(11): 6123.
17. Larsen CP, Morris PJ and Austyn JM. Migration of dendritic leukocytes from cardiac allografts into host spleens. A novel pathway for initiation of rejection. *J Exp Med* 1990; 171(1): 307.
18. Game DS and Lechler RI. Pathways of allorecognition: implications for transplantation tolerance. *Transpl Immunol* 2002; 10(2–3): 101.
19. Kurts C *et al.* Dendritic cells are sufficient to cross-present self-antigens to CD8 T cells *in vivo*. *J Immunol* 2001; 166(3): 1439.
20. Starzl TE and Demetris AJ. Transplantation tolerance, microchimerism, and the two-way paradigm. *Theor Med Bioeth* 1998; 19(5): 441.
21. Streilein JW, Toews GB and Bergstresser PR. Corneal allografts fail to express Ia antigens. *Nature* 1979; 282(5736): 326.
22. Whitsett CF and Stulting RD. The distribution of HLA antigens on human corneal tissue. *Invest Ophthalmol Vis Sci* 1984; 25(5): 519.
23. Benichou G, Valujskikh A and Heeger PS. Contributions of direct and indirect T cell alloreactivity during allograft rejection in mice. *J Immunol* 1999; 162(1): 352.
24. Millrain M *et al.* Examination of HY response: T cell expansion, immunodominance, and cross-priming revealed by HY tetramer analysis. *J Immunol* 2001; 167(7): 3756.
25. Bingaman AW *et al.* Vigorous allograft rejection in the absence of danger. *J Immunol* 2000; 164(6): 3065.
26. Sano Y, Ksander BR and Streilein JW. Minor H, rather than MHC, alloantigens offer the greater barrier to successful orthotopic corneal transplantation in mice. *Transpl Immunol* 1996; 4(1): 53.
27. Rolls HK *et al.* T-cell response to cardiac myosin persists in the absence of an alloimmune response in recipients with chronic cardiac allograft rejection. *Transplantation* 2002; 74(7): 1053.
28. Valujskikh A *et al.* Development of autoimmunity after skin graft rejection via an indirect alloresponse. *Transplantation* 2002; 73(7): 1130.
29. Liu Z *et al.* Contribution of direct and indirect recognition pathways to T cell alloreactivity. *J Exp Med* 1993; 177(6): 1643.
30. Kuffová L *et al.* Kinetics of leukocyte and myeloid cell traffic in the murine corneal allograft response. *Transplantation* 2001; 72(7): 1292.
31. He YG and Niederkorn JY. Depletion of donor-derived Langerhans cells promotes corneal allograft survival. *Cornea* 1996; 15(1): 82.
32. Liu Y *et al.* Draining lymph nodes of corneal transplant hosts exhibit evidence for donor major histocompatibility complex (MHC) class II-positive dendritic cells derived from MHC class II-negative grafts. *J Exp Med* 2002; 195(2): 259.
33. Bradley BA *et al.* Negative effect of HLA-DR matching on corneal transplant rejection. *Transplant Proc* 1995; 27(1): 1392.
34. Nicholls SM and Williams NA. MHC matching and mechanisms of alloactivation in corneal transplantation. *Transplantation* 2001; 72(9): 1491.
35. Volker-Dieben HJ *et al.* Beneficial effect of HLA-DR matching on the survival of corneal allografts. *Transplantation* 2000; 70(4): 640.

36. Fox-Marsh A and Harrison LC. Emerging evidence that molecules expressed by mammalian tissue grafts are recognized by the innate immune system. *J Leukoc Biol* 2002; 71(3): 401.
37. Plšková J *et al.* Evaluation of corneal graft rejection in a mouse model. *Br J Ophthalmol* 2002; 86(1): 108.
38. Yamagami S and Tsuru T. Increase in orthotopic murine corneal transplantation rejection rate with anterior synechiae. *Invest Ophthalmol Vis Sci* 1999; 40(10): 2422.
39. Hegde S *et al.* Effect of alloantibodies on corneal allograft survival. *Invest Ophthalmol Vis Sci* 2002; 43(4): 1012.
40. Hargrave SL *et al.* High-risk corneal allografts are capable of stimulating complement dependent cytolytic antibodies. *Cornea* 2000; 19(4): 521.
41. Goslings WR *et al.* Corneal transplantation in antibody-deficient hosts. *Invest Ophthalmol Vis Sci* 1999; 40(1): 250.
42. Reinhard T *et al.* Immune cells in the anterior chamber of patients with immune reactions after penetrating keratoplasty. *Cornea* 2002; 21(1): 56.
43. Kuffová L *et al.* Cell subpopulations in failed human corneal grafts. *Br J Ophthalmol* 1999; 83(12): 1364.
44. Larkin DF, Alexander RA and Cree IA. Infiltrating inflammatory cell phenotypes and apoptosis in rejected human corneal allografts. *Eye* 1997; 11(Pt 1): 68.
45. Larkin DF, Calder VL and Lightman SL. Identification and characterization of cells infiltrating the graft and aqueous humour in rat corneal allograft rejection. *Clin Exp Immunol* 1997; 107(2): 381.
46. Krause L, Coupland SE and Hoffmann F. The behaviour of ED1- and ED2-positive cells in the rat iris and choroid following penetrating keratoplasty and cyclosporin A therapy. *Graefes Arch Clin Exp Ophthalmol* 1996; 234 Suppl 1: S149.
47. Torres PF *et al.* Cytokine mRNA expression during experimental corneal allograft rejection. *Exp Eye Res* 1996; 63(4): 453.
48. Takano T and Williams KA. Mechanism of corneal endothelial destruction in rejecting rat corneal allografts and xenografts: a role for CD4+ cells. *Transplant Proc* 1995; 27(1): 260.
49. Coupland S, Billson F and Hoffmann F. Hydrolase participation in allograft rejection in rat penetrating keratoplasty. *Graefes Arch Clin Exp Ophthalmol* 1994; 232(10): 614.
50. Holland EJ *et al.* Kinetics of corneal transplant rejection in the rat penetrating keratoplasty model. *Cornea* 1994; 13(4): 317.
51. Holland EJ *et al.* Clinical and immunohistologic studies of corneal rejection in the rat penetrating keratoplasty model. *Cornea* 1991; 10(5): 374.
52. Goldberg MF, Ferguson TA and Pepose JS. Detection of cellular adhesion molecules in inflamed human corneas. *Ophthalmology* 1994; 101(1): 161.
53. Polack FM. The endothelium of failed corneal grafts. *Am J Ophthalmol* 1975; 79(2): 251.
54. Gebhardt BM. Cell-mediated immunity in the cornea. *Transplantation* 1988; 46(2): 273.
55. Slegers TP *et al.* Delayed graft rejection in pre-vascularised corneas after subconjunctival injection of clodronate liposomes. *Curr Eye Res* 2000; 20(4): 322.
56. Slegers TP *et al.* Effect of macrophage depletion on immune effector mechanisms during corneal allograft rejection in rats. *Invest Ophthalmol Vis Sci* 2000; 41(8): 2239.
57. Warren HS and Smyth MJ. NK cells and apoptosis. *Immunol Cell Biol* 1999; 77(1): 64.

58. Petersson E *et al.* Allogeneic heart transplantation activates alloreactive NK cells. *Cell Immunol* 1997; 175(1): 25.
59. He H, Stone JR and Perkins DL. Analysis of robust innate immune response after transplantation in the absence of adaptive immunity. *Transplantation* 2002; 73(6): 853.
60. Brissette-Storkus CS *et al.* Identification of a novel macrophage population in the normal mouse corneal stroma. *Invest Ophthalmol Vis Sci* 2002; 43(7): 2264.
61. Apte RS and Niederkorn JY. Isolation and characterization of a unique natural killer cell inhibitory factor present in the anterior chamber of the eye. *J Immunol* 1996; 156(8): 2667.
62. Apte RS *et al.* Cutting edge: role of macrophage migration inhibitory factor in inhibiting NK cell activity and preserving immune privilege. *J Immunol* 1998; 160(12): 5693.
63. Fernandez NC *et al.* Dendritic cells directly trigger NK cell functions: cross-talk relevant in innate anti-tumor immune responses *in vivo. Nat Med* 1999; 5(4): 405.
64. Moretta A. Natural killer cells and dendritic cells: rendezvous in abused tissues. *Nat Rev Immunol* 2002; 2(12): 957.
65. Callanan DG *et al.* Histopathology of rejected orthotopic corneal grafts in the rat. *Invest Ophthalmol Vis Sci* 1989; 30(3): 413.
66. Dekaris I, Zhu SN and Dana MR. TNF-alpha regulates corneal Langerhans cell migration. *J Immunol* 1999; 162(7): 4235.
67. Hamrah P *et al.* Novel characterization of MHC class II-negative population of resident corneal Langerhans cell-type dendritic cells. *Invest Ophthalmol Vis Sci* 2002; 43(3): 639.
68. Hori J, Joyce NC and Streilein JW. Immune privilege and immunogenicity reside among different layers of the mouse cornea. *Invest Ophthalmol Vis Sci* 2000; 41(10): 3032.
69. Hori J and Streilein JW. Role of recipient epithelium in promoting survival of orthotopic corneal allografts in mice. *Invest Ophthalmol Vis Sci* 2001; 42(3): 720.
70. Niederkorn JY. The immune privilege of corneal allografts. *Transplantation* 1999; 67(12): 1503.
71. Sano Y, Ksander BR and Streilein JW. Langerhans cells, orthotopic corneal allografts, and direct and indirect pathways of T-cell allorecognition. *Invest Ophthalmol Vis Sci* 2000; 41(6): 1422.
72 Williams KA and Coster DJ. The role of the limbus in corneal allograft rejection. *Eye* 1989; 3(Pt 2): 158.
73. Niederkorn JY. Immune privilege in the anterior chamber of the eye. *Crit Rev Immunol* 2002; 22(1): 13.
74. Egan RM *et al.* Peptide-specific T cell clonal expansion *in vivo* following immunization in the eye, an immune-privileged site. *J Immunol* 1996; 157(6): 2262.
75. Hoffmann F *et al.* Contribution of lymphatic drainage system in corneal allograft rejection in mice. *Graefes Arch Clin Exp Ophthalmol* 2001; 239(11): 850.
76. Yatoh S *et al.* Effect of a topically applied neutralizing antibody against vascular endothelial growth factor on corneal allograft rejection of rat. *Transplantation* 1998; 66(11): 1519.
77. Gebhardt BM and Seto SK. The immunogenicity of corneal stromal keratocytes. *Transplantation* 1988; 46(3): 444.
78. Boisgerault F *et al.* Role of CD4+ and CD8+ T cells in allorecognition: lessons from corneal transplantation. *J Immunol*, 2001; 167(4): 1891.

79. Hašková Z *et al.* CD4+ T cells are critical for corneal, but not skin, allograft rejection. *Transplantation* 2000; 69(4): 483.
80. He YG, Ross J and Niederkorn JY. Promotion of murine orthotopic corneal allograft survival by systemic administration of anti-CD4 monoclonal antibody. *Invest Ophthalmol Vis Sci* 1991; 32(10): 2723.
81. Bingaman AW *et al.* Analysis of the CD40 and CD28 pathways on alloimmune responses by CD4+ T cells *in vivo. Transplantation* 2001; 72(7): 1286.
82. Jonker M *et al.* Blocking the CD80 and CD86 costimulation molecules: lessons to be learned from animal models. *Transplantation* 2002; 73(1 Suppl): S23.
83. Rifle G and Mousson C. Dendritic cells and second signal blockade: a step toward allograft tolerance? *Transplantation* 2002; 73(1 Suppl): S1.
84. Qian Y and Dana MR. Effect of locally administered anti-CD154 (CD40 ligand) monoclonal antibody on survival of allogeneic corneal transplants. *Cornea* 2002; 21(6): 592.
85. Frauwirth KA and Thompson CB. Activation and inhibition of lymphocytes by costimulation. *J Clin Invest* 2002; 109(3): 295.
86. Greenwald RJ, Latchman YE and Sharpe AH. Negative co-receptors on lymphocytes. *Curr Opin Immunol* 2002; 14(3): 391.
87. Prilliman KR *et al.* Cutting edge: a crucial role for B7-CD28 in transmitting T help from APC to CTL. *J Immunol* 2002; 169(8): 4094.
88. Hodi FS *et al.* Biologic activity of cytotoxic T lymphocyte-associated antigen 4 antibody blockade in previously vaccinated metastatic melanoma and ovarian carcinoma patients. *Proc Natl Acad Sci USA* 2003; 100(8): 4712.
89. Egen JG, Kuhns MS and Allison JP. CTLA-4: new insights into its biological function and use in tumor immunotherapy. *Nat Immunol* 2002; 3(7): 611.
90. Jenkins MK *et al. In vivo* activation of antigen-specific CD4 T cells. *Annu Rev Immunol* 2001; 19: 23.
91. Ingulli E *et al. In situ* analysis reveals physical interactions between CD11b+ dendritic cells and antigen-specific CD4 T cells after subcutaneous injection of antigen. *J Immunol* 2002; 169(5): 2247.
92. Williams KA *et al.* A new model of orthotopic penetrating corneal transplantation in the sheep: graft survival, phenotypes of graft-infiltrating cells and local cytokine production. *Aust N Z J Ophthalmol* 1999; 27(2): 127.
93. King WJ *et al.* Cytokine and chemokine expression kinetics after corneal transplantation. *Transplantation* 2000; 70(8): 1225.
94. Luster AD. The role of chemokines in linking innate and adaptive immunity. *Curr Opin Immunol* 2002; 14(1): 129.
95. Caux C *et al.* Regulation of dendritic cell recruitment by chemokines. *Transplantation* 2002; 73(1 Suppl): S7.
96. Hori J *et al.* Specific immunosuppression of corneal allograft rejection by combination of anti-VLA-4 and anti-LFA-1 monoclonal antibodies in mice. *Exp Eye Res* 1997; 65(1): 89.
97. Yamagami S, Isobe M and Tsuru T. Characterization of cytokine profiles in corneal allograft with anti-adhesion therapy. *Transplantation* 2000; 69(8): 1655.
98. Yamada J, Kurimoto I and Streilein JW. Role of CD4+ T cells in immunobiology of orthotopic corneal transplants in mice. *Invest Ophthalmol Vis Sci* 1999; 40(11): 2614.

99. Yamada J, Ksander BR and Streilein JW. Cytotoxic T cells play no essential role in acute rejection of orthotopic corneal allografts in mice. *Invest Ophthalmol Vis Sci* 2001; 42(2): 386.
100. Peeler J, Niederkorn J and Matoba A. Corneal allografts induce cytotoxic T cell but not delayed hypersensitivity responses in mice. *Invest Ophthalmol Vis Sci* 1985; 26(11): 1516.
101. Joo CK, Pepose JS and Stuart PM. T-cell mediated responses in a murine model of orthotopic corneal transplantation. *Invest Ophthalmol Vis Sci* 1995; 36(8): 1530.
102. Hegde S and Niederkorn JY. The role of cytotoxic T lymphocytes in corneal allograft rejection. *Invest Ophthalmol Vis Sci* 2000; 41(11): 3341.
103. Miura M *et al.* Monokine induced by IFN-gamma is a dominant factor directing T cells into murine cardiac allografts during acute rejection. *J Immunol* 2001; 167(6): 3494.
104. Cua DJ *et al.* Interleukin-23 rather than interleukin-12 is the critical cytokine for autoimmune inflammation of the brain. *Nature* 2003; 421(6924): 744.
105. Borish LC and Steinke JW. 2. Cytokines and chemokines. *J Allergy Clin Immunol* 2003; 111(2 Suppl): S460.
106. Yun JJ *et al.* The role of MIG/CXCL9 in cardiac allograft vasculopathy. *Am J Pathol* 2002; 161(4): 1307.
107. Ferguson TA *et al.* Uptake of apoptotic antigen-coupled cells by lymphoid dendritic cells and cross-priming of CD8(+) T cells produce active immune unresponsiveness. *J Immunol* 2002; 168(11): 5589.
108. Hori J and Streilein JW. Dynamics of donor cell persistence and recipient cell replacement in orthotopic corneal allografts in mice. *Invest Ophthalmol Vis Sci* 2001; 42(8): 1820.
109. Brent L *et al.* Transplantation tolerance. *Br Med Bull* 1976; 32(2): 101.
110. Niederkorn J, Streilein JW and Shadduck JA. Deviant immune responses to allogeneic tumors injected intracamerally and subcutaneously in mice. *Invest Ophthalmol Vis Sci* 1981; 20(3): 355.
111. Kaplan HJ and Streilein JW. Analysis of immunologic privilege within the anterior chamber of the eye. *Transplant Proc* 1977; 9(1): 1193.
112. Kaplan HJ and Streilein JW. Immune response to immunization via the anterior chamber of the eye. II. An analysis of F1 lymphocyte-induced immune deviation. *J Immunol* 1978; 120(3): 689.
113. Ditzian-Kadanoff R. Testicular-associated immune deviation and prevention of adjuvant-induced arthritis by three tolerization methods. *Scand J Immunol* 1999; 50(2): 150.
114. Wenkel H, Streilein JW and Young MJ. Systemic immune deviation in the brain that does not depend on the integrity of the blood-brain barrier. *J Immunol* 2000; 164(10): 5125.
115. Verdaguer J *et al.* Two mechanisms for the non-MHC-linked resistance to spontaneous autoimmunity. *J Immunol* 1999; 162(8): 4614.
116. Streilein JW. Ocular immune privilege and the Faustian dilemma. The Proctor Lecture. *Invest Ophthalmol Vis Sci* 1996; 37(10): 1940.
117. McMenamin PG. Dendritic cells and macrophages in the uveal tract of the normal mouse eye. *Br J Ophthalmol* 1999; 83(5): 598.
118. McMenamin PG. Distribution and phenotype of dendritic cells and resident tissue macrophages in the dura mater, leptomeninges, and choroid plexus of the rat brain as demonstrated in wholemount preparations. *J Comp Neurol* 1999; 405(4): 553.

119. McMenamin PG. The distribution of immune cells in the uveal tract of the normal eye. *Eye* 1997; 11 (Pt 2): 183.
120. Steptoe RJ, Holt PG and McMenamin PG. Functional studies of major histocompatibility class II-positive dendritic cells and resident tissue macrophages isolated from the rat iris. *Immunology* 1995; 85(4): 630.
121. McMenamin PG *et al.* Immunomorphologic studies of macrophages and MHC class II-positive dendritic cells in the iris and ciliary body of the rat, mouse, and human eye. *Invest Ophthalmol Vis Sci* 1994; 35(8): 3234.
122. Forrester JV *et al.* Localization and characterization of major histocompatibility complex class II-positive cells in the posterior segment of the eye: implications for induction of autoimmune uveoretinitis. *Invest Ophthalmol Vis Sci* 1994; 35(1): 64.
123. Cross AK and Woodroofe MN. Immunoregulation of microglial functional properties. *Microsc Res Tech* 2001; 54(1): 10.
124. Griffith TS *et al.* Fas ligand-induced apoptosis as a mechanism of immune privilege. *Science* 1995; 270(5239): 1189.
125. Griffith TS *et al.* CD95-induced apoptosis of lymphocytes in an immune privileged site induces immunological tolerance. *Immunity* 1996; 5(1): 7.
126. Lee HO *et al.* TRAIL: a mechanism of tumor surveillance in an immune privileged site. *J Immunol* 2002; 169(9): 4739.
127. Gregory MS *et al.* Membrane Fas ligand activates innate immunity and terminates ocular immune privilege. *J Immunol* 2002; 169(5): 2727.
128. Green DR and Ferguson TA. The role of Fas ligand in immune privilege. *Nat Rev Mol Cell Biol* 2001; 2(12): 917.
129. She SC and Moticka EJ. Ability of intracamerally inoculated B- and T-cell enriched allogeneic lymphocytes to enhance corneal allograft survival. *Int Ophthalmol* 1993; 17(1): 1.
130. She SC, Steahly LP and Moticka EJ. Intracameral injection of allogeneic lymphocytes enhances corneal graft survival. *Invest Ophthalmol Vis Sci 1990;* 31(10): 1950.
131. Stein-Streilein J and Streilein JW. Anterior chamber associated immune deviation (ACAID): regulation, biological relevance, and implications for therapy. *Int Rev Immunol* 2002; 21(2–3): 123.
132. Wang Y *et al.* Blood mononuclear cells induce regulatory NK T thymocytes in anterior chamber-associated immune deviation. *J Leukoc Biol* 2001; 69(5): 741.
133. Plšková J *et al.* The immune response to corneal allograft requires a site-specific draining lymph node. Transplantation 2002; 73(2): 210.
134. Dutton RW, Bradley LM and Swain SL. T cell memory. *Annu Rev Immunol* 1998; 16: 201.
135. Akbari O *et al.* DNA vaccination: transfection and activation of dendritic cells as key events for immunity. *J Exp Med* 1999; 189(1): 169.
136. He YG *et al.* Acceptance of H-Y-disparate corneal grafts despite concomitant immunization of the recipient. *Transplantation* 1991; 51(6): 1258.
137. He YG, Mellon J and Niederkorn JY. The effect of oral immunization on corneal allograft survival. *Transplantation* 1996; 61(6): 920.
138. Ma D, Mellon J and Niederkorn JY. Oral immunisation as a strategy for enhancing corneal allograft survival. *Br J Ophthalmol* 1997; 81(9): 778.

139. Ma D, Mellon J and Niederkorn JY. Conditions affecting enhanced corneal allograft survival by oral immunization. *Invest Ophthalmol Vis Sci* 1998; 39(10):1835.
140. Weiner HL. Oral tolerance: immune mechanisms and the generation of Th3-type TGF-beta-secreting regulatory cells. *Microbes Infect* 2001; 3(11): 947.
141. Holáň V *et al.* Induction of specific transplantation immunity by oral immunization with allogeneic cells. *Immunology* 2000; 101(3): 404.
142. Waldmann H and Cobbold S. Approaching tolerance in transplantation. *Int Arch Allergy Immunol* 2001; 126(1): 11.
143. Bluestone JA and Abbas AK. Natural versus adaptive regulatory T cells. *Nat Rev Immunol* 2003; 3(3): 253.
144. DePaz HA *et al.* Immature rat myeloid dendritic cells generated in low-dose granulocyte macrophage-colony stimulating factor prolong donor-specific rat cardiac allograft survival. *Transplantation* 2003; 75(4): 521.
145. Solomon A and Frucht-Pery J. Bilateral simultaneous corneal graft rejection after influenza vaccination. *Am J Ophthalmol* 1996; 121(6): 708.

7

The Xenoresponse to Corneal Graft

Introduction

Xenotransplantation is a long-cherished notion for solving the problem of the scarcity of organ donor supply while providing the physiological functions of vital organs [1]. Questions of phylogeny have not presented an intellectual barrier to the concept: lamellar chicken corneal grafts remain clear in rabbits [2] and as recently as 1973, fish corneas were being proposed as possible xenografts for humans [3]. However, the difficulties presented by immune rejection of allografts are magnified several fold by the rapid rejection of xenotransplants and there are several mechanisms underlying this process. For vascularized xenografts there are in addition many physiological and anatomic incompatibilities which add further complexity to the acceptance of a graft [4]. Some of these also apply to the cornea. Many difficulties therefore require to be overcome before this technology can become a realistic possibility, and approaches such as generating biohybrid xenotransplants with human stem cells are under consideration [5].

Xenotransplantation of the cornea has a long history, predating the emergence of immunology itself as a scientific discipline by several decades: one of the earliest corneal transplants to a human was from a donor pig (see Chapter 1) but, as might be expected, this was not successful. However, the study of xenotransplantation of the cornea has an important contribution to make to our understanding of the immunology of xenorejection since the avascular cornea cannot generate the acute vascular response which is the hallmark for rejection of other solid organ xenotransplants. Corneal xenotransplants are still rejected, however, and thus provide information on the several other mechanisms at play.

The Immune Response to Xenografts

The most immediate perceived need for xenotransplantation derives from the lack of human donor vital organs such as heart, kidney and liver all of which are vascularized. The immune response to these xenografts is predominantly directed towards the blood vessels and is very rapid. Several pathological processes are entrained during the rejection of xenografts and they occur at different rates: hyperacute rejection (HAR) takes place classically within minutes to hours but may be delayed beyond 24 hours; acute rejection, also called acute vascular rejection (AVR), which occurs in vascularized solid organ grafts that may have survived HAR; mixed delayed HAR and acute rejection; and chronic rejection (graft arteriopathy) [6]. In addition, there is a process termed "accommodation" in which xenografts protected from rejection by depletion of "natural" antibodies, appear to survive rejection when the level of these antibodies returns to normal.

Many cells and molecules are involved, most of which would be included within the innate immune defence network but adaptive responses also occur although at a much reduced level.

Cells and molecules in the xenograft response

Several different mechanisms may be involved in xenogrft rejection but the rapidity of rejection indicates that many of the molecules and cells are preformed. Complement (C) proteins are central to the acute response and both the classical and the alternative pathways may be involved. The normal regulation of the alternative pathway by Factor H, through inhibition of C3b by factor B, is lacking across some species, while in others the classical pathway is activated by "natural" C1q-fixing antibodies. In addition, other complement regulatory proteins such as CD55, 46 and 59 function in a species-specific manner and thus may not be available to protect against complement attack in a xenograft. This is particularly relevant to the eye where C regulatory proteins are important components of immune privilege [7–11] and the transgenic expression of human C regulatory proteins in pigs may help to overcome this problem. "Natural" antibodies are so called because they exist in the circulation without any previous exposure to foreign antigens. They are of two types: antibodies against specific carbohydrate antigens, the best known of which are the anti-Galα1,3Gal antibodies and the antibodies to blood group antigens; and antibodies which react against a range of surface structures but are of low affinity and therefore less immunogenic. Galα1,3Gal is a carbohydrate present in many lower mammals such as pigs but not humans and antibodies in humans are thought to arise during the first years of life due to cross-reactive gut bacterial colonisation [12].

Most inflammatory cells are involved in the immune response to xenotransplantation including neutrophils, macrophages, T cells and NK cells [13]. In addition, intravascular and tissue blood/plasma clotting is a prominent feature of the xenograft response involving extensive thrombin and platelet activation [14]. Neutrophils are involved via complement activation but may also have a direct effect in causing endothelial cell damage. NK cells may exert their effect via failure of xeno-MHC Class I to inhibit their action. They are probably also activated directly by IgG-FcγII interactions as well as through Galα1,3Gal-lectin receptors on NK cells [15]. T cells have a limited response mediated via an "indirect" pathway of xenoantigen presentation to host APC and there is even some evidence for a "direct" response to foreign MHC in this instance [16].

Coagulation is induced by spontaneous thrombin activation, e.g. on pig endothelium, and this is thought to be due once more to cross-species failure of regulatory molecules such as thrombomodulin [17]. Activation of thrombin then leads to platelet activation and amplification of the coagulation process via tissue factor release, E/P selectin upregulation and inflammatory cell adhesion to the endothelium.

Hyperacute rejection (HAR)

HAR is directed against blood vessels and the severity of the response is determined by the origin of the graft vessels [18]. Skin grafts may be composed of a mixture of host and donor anastomotic vessels, while larger organs such as the heart and kidney require survival of donor vessels for physiological functioning. HAR is instant and causes graft failure within hours; it is due to the activation of complement on the endothelium (see above). If activation occurs through the alternative pathway it is intense whereas if it occurs via natural antibodies the tempo of rejection is a little slower. Complement activation through this mechanism is not of itself cytotoxic but causes endothelial cell retraction and loss of vessel integrity. If complement activation can be inhibited or delayed, the xenograft may survive this initial event.

The major natural antibody which activates complement in this situation is anti-Galα1,3Gal, which accounts for about 1% of immunoglobulins in human plasma [19].

Xenotransplantation to primates of kidneys from pigs which were genetically modified to express the human complement inhibitor, decay accelerating factor (hDAF) were shown to have a reduced incidence of HAR and a prolonged (but still brief, i.e. up to four days) survival [20]. Thus while there is some progress in preventing HAR, many problems of acute and chronic rejection remain.

Acute (vascular) rejection

Strategies which bypass complement activation in xenografts delay but do not prevent rejection. In vascularized grafts rejection is manifested by endothelial cell damage and intravascular coagulation which develops over days to weeks. Recent studies have indicated that the venous component of the circulatory loop is particularly susceptible to this form of rejection and that capillaries become damaged by the expanding back pressure from the occluded veins [21]. Platelets, macrophages and NK cells appear to be intimately involved in this process but usually as a late event and then by causing cell damage. Direct activation of procoagulant molecules by the endothelium is considered less likely than induction by antibodies reacting against xenoantigens on the graft principally anti-Galα1,3Gal but also other antibodies.

Interestingly, some xenografts can survive antibody-mediated attack if there is initial depletion, e.g. of blood group antibodies, even when these antibodies return to normal levels after some time. This process is termed accommodation but the precise mechanisms is unknown [22]. It appears to be associated with the production of antiapoptotic molecules and other more general molecular pathways, such as heme oxygenase-1 and ferritin [23].

Chronic rejection

Evidence for chronic rejection in xenografts is difficult to obtain. In the pig to human xenograft system, elimination of the Gal antigen would appear to be essential in order to determine the amount of non-HAR and nonacute rejection would be responsible ultimately for failure of any given graft [24] but development of such Tg pigs has proved elusive, possible because Gal antigen is essential to the pig. Recent studies in Tg Gal KO mice have shown that the Gal mismatch alone can cause rejection which is usually chronic [25] and which could be accelerated if the animals were passively immunized with anti-Gal antibodies.

Role of the innate immune system in rejection of xenografts

Most of the effects of the immune response to vascularized xenografts appear to be mediated via innate immune mechanisms. Despite the fact that "natural" antibodies, by definition produced adaptively by B cells/plasma cells responding to cross reactive galactosyl-containing residues in bacterial antigenic epitopes from gut commensals, the final common pathway is unregulated activation of complement and extensive endothelial cell damage [6]. This induces the recruitment of cells of the innate immune system.

The innate immune response to nonvascularized grafts such as pancreatic islets is somewhat different. It has previously been shown that macrophages, including a subset which expresses CD4, are important mediators of the innate immune response to pancreatic xenografts [26] and more recent studies have shown that the PAMPs (see Chapter 6) involved in both xenografts and to a lesser extent in allografts are probably oligosaccharides on the surface of donor cells [27]. Blood group antigens are a possible source for these responses [28].

The Immune Response to Corneal Xenografts

There has been no lack of imagination in developing experimental models of xenotransplantation for the cornea. For instance, a corneal defect after excision of a melanoma has been successfully repaired using a pig xenograft of small intestine submucosa [29]. More conventionally, both large animal (human to cat!) [30] and small animal [31, 32] orthotopic corneal xenograft models have been developed and for the same general reasons as for allografts, i.e. large animal models are designed to examine specific aspects of corneal pathophysiology during rejection and small animal models are generally directed towards investigation of immune mechanisms of rejection (see Chapter 8). In addition, study of specific cell function has been addressed for instance in the use of nude mice as hosts for human limbal stem cells after culture on amniotic membrane [33] and transplantation of autologous corneas on which cultured heterologous endothelial cells had previously been grown [34]. Heterologous amniotic membrane itself appears not to induce a significant immune response [35].

The immune response to corneal xenografts

Corneal xenograft rejection requires transplantation of live cells: bovine cell-free lyophilized and reconstituted lamellar grafts placed into the rabbit stroma do not induce an immune response and remain clear [36].

The immunology of rejection of live corneal xenotransplants is significantly different from vascularized organ xenotransplants. Firstly, as for other nonvascularized grafts such as cultured fetal pig pancreatic islets [26], HAR does not occur [32]. Second, xenotransplanted corneas do not enjoy the privilege of corneal allografts since irreversible rejection occurs in all cases [31] and fragments of xenogeneic cornea placed in the anterior chamber do not induce immune deviation [37]. The processes involved in this delayed yet nonprivileged rejection are unknown but are likely to involve the secondary mechanisms entrained in vascularized xenograft rejection when HAR is experimentally blocked. These include xenoreactive antibodies, NK cells and macrophages [38–40]. In addition, chronic rejection, also known as cell-mediated rejection and involving T cells, may play a part if both HAR and acute (delayed) rejection are prevented [41].

Previous studies of corneal xenografts between guinea pigs and rats have shown that clinical graft rejection occurs around 8–9 days and can be accelerated if the animals are presensitized to xenoantigen [42, 43]. Other studies have shown that rejection can occur as early as day 3 [31] but the HAR response of minutes to hours is not evident in this system. Histological studies, however, reveal that at the earliest point studied after grafting, infiltrates of macrophages and neutrophils are present in the posterior corneal stroma and immunohistology revealed the presence of a significant infiltrate of T cells [43]. Therefore although clinical rejection is not evident for some days, there is a very early innate, and possibly a developing adaptive immune response if this is relevant to xenograft rejection. In fact an early study of corneal xenografts in rats indicated that CD4+ T cells may play an active role [44]. There is also the likelihood that humoral mechanisms play a role since extensive deposition of IgG and IgM antibody was present in the stroma [43] and graft rejection occurred even when the xenografts were placed into immunodeficient rats [31].

Tanaka *et al.* investigated the immunological responses further using a guinea pig to mouse model. Remarkably, they showed that prolonged survival (>8 weeks) of clear guinea pig grafts could be obtained in immunodeficient mice in whom a protective tarsorrhaphy had also been performed to prevent chronic ocular surface damage due to protrusion of the thick guinea pig cornea placed in the mouse cornea [45]. In immunocompetent mice guinea pig corneas remained clear for 10 days (H-2^b) or 16 days (H-2^d); the histology showed an extensively swollen graft with massive cellular infiltration and loss of both epithelium and endothelium. Using a range of knockout mice, it was shown that neither antibody/B cells, CD8+ T cells or NKT cells were required for acute rejection whereas CD4+ T cells were necessary. In addition, there was a minor role for complement. Delayed rejection still occurred in CD4KO mice and this element of chronic rejection may in part be due to CD8+ T cell–mediated mechanisms. Further investigation showed that chronic rejection was indeed due predominantly to the effect of CD8+ T cells [46], indicating a significant mechanistic difference from corneal allograft rejection where CD8+ T cells play little part (see Chapter 6). However, there also appear to be additional as yet undefined mechanisms involved in corneal xenograft rejection [46]. A role for the adaptive immune response on xenograft rejection can be inferred from data indicating that the immunosuppressive agent, FK 506 can delay rejection [47], although this drug may also have more direct effects on leukocyte–endothelial cell interactions [48].

The adaptive immune response to corneal xenografts appears to occur almost exclusively by the "indirect" route [49], i.e. the conventional route for presentation of foreign antigen to T cells via host antigen-presenting cells. In this experiment, guinea pig corneal grafts survived for a prolonged time in mice deficient in MHC Class II, who are also deficient in T cells. Reconstitution with naïve T cells alone or with antigen-presenting cells alone failed to restore the normal tempo of rejection. However, the effect of reconstitution with xenoantigen primed T cells was not tested and might have provided some further information on the precise role of T cells in this process. Even though there is likely to be a population of passenger leukocytes in xenogeneic corneas [50], they are unlikely to be involved in direct xenoantigen presentation to host T cells since this mechanisms is not invoked for any type of xenograft response. Interestingly, both human corneal epithelium and skin epidermis fail to express reactivity against anti-αGal antibodies, unlike other epithelial layers [51]. In addition, aqueous contains anticomplement activity although this is clearly insufficient to inhibit xenograft rejection [52].

The Use of Corneal Xenografts to Study Human Corneal Wound Healing

There is intense current interest in the physiology of wound healing in the human cornea due to the widespread developments in refractive surgery [53–55]. Histological studies of the early stages of wound healing in the human cornea have been made possible by the xenotransplantation of human corneas to cats and have been justified on the basis that the HAR does not occur in the cornea [30, 56]. In the rat to guinea pig the immune response is reported not to develop until eight days after grafting [42, 43] while in the human to monkey, corneal graft rejection does not occur until four months have passed [57]. However, these assumptions may be ill-founded. It has been shown in corneal allografting that the innate immune response is initiated within hours of graft emplacement and that there is recruitment of T cells to the cornea within 24–48 hours (see Chapter 6). In addition, the innate immune response to xenografts is recognized to be very powerful even in the absence of complement-mediated mechanisms which is the basis of HAR. Therefore, it is likely that the keratocyte activation and apoptosis seen in the human to cat model during the early stages of wound healing [30, 56] are taking place against a background of an ongoing strong immune response and may even be contributing to the cell death. The results of these experiments therefore require to be interpreted cautiously.

Possible Systemic Complications of Xenografts

Currently there are no successful long term accepted xenografts. Considerable effort is currently being expended in developing transgenic animals, particularly pigs for use as sources of solid organ xenografts. Difficulties in deleting the Gal gene have already been referred to above but other genes may also have to be targeted if the various mechanisms of graft rejection are to be overcome. However, newer more efficient techniques for genetic modification are required before large scale success in pigs can be achieved [58].

This raises the possibility of risk from genetically modified animals. At present the risk is unquantified and much of the discussion around this issue is theoretical. However, safeguards are required.

Conclusion

Use of corneal xenografts is attractive for several reasons but particularly because of the shortage of available donor corneas. Successful acceptance of corneas is more likely than for other xenografts due to the lack of the HAR response. For immunologists this also offers the interesting possibility of investigation of the later immune responses to xenografts without having to intervene to prevent HAR.

References

1. Rocha H and Gustavo Galvao P. Immunological aspects of corneal heterografts. *Int Ophthalmol Clin* 1966; 6(1): 19.
2. D'Ermo F, Lanzieri M and Revoltella R. Effects of a passive administration of humoral antibodies, sensitized polymorpholeukocytes and immunologically competent lymphocytes in rabbits supporting transparent inter-lamellar chicken corneal grafts. *Acta Ophthalmol (Copenh)* 1969; 47(4): 822.
3. Haq M. Fish cornea for grafting. *Br Med J* 1972; 2(815): 712.
4. Hammer C and Thein E. Physiological aspects of xenotransplantation 2001. *Xenotransplantation* 2002; 9(5): 303.
5. Brasile L, Stubenitsky BM and Kootstra G. Solving the organ shortage: potential strategies and the likelihood of success. *Asaio J* 2002; 48(3): 211.
6. Cascalho M and Platt JL. The immunological barrier to xenotransplantation. *Immunity* 2001; 14(4): 437.
7. Liversidge J *et al.* CD59 and CD48 expressed by rat retinal pigment epithelial cells are major ligands for the CD2-mediated alternative pathway of T cell activation. *J Immunol* 1996; 156(10): 3696.
8. Sohn JH *et al.* Chronic low level complement activation within the eye is controlled by intraocular complement regulatory proteins. *Invest Ophthalmol Vis Sci* 2000; 41(11): 3492.
9. Sohn JH *et al.* Complement regulatory activity of normal human intraocular fluid is mediated by MCP, DAF, and CD59. *Invest Ophthalmol Vis Sci* 2000; 41(13): 4195.
10. Sohn JH *et al.* Tolerance is dependent on complement C3 fragment iC3b binding to antigen-presenting cells. *Nat Med* 2003; 9(2): 206.
11. Bora NS *et al.* Differential expression of the complement regulatory proteins in the human eye. *Invest Ophthalmol Vis Sci* 1993; 34(13): 3579.
12. Tucker A *et al.* The production of transgenic pigs for potential use in clinical xenotransplantation: microbiological evaluation. *Xenotransplantation* 2002; 9(3): 191.

13. Holgersson J *et al.* Leukocyte endothelial cell interactions in pig to human organ xenograft rejection. *Vet Immunol Immunopathol* 2002; 87(3–4): 407.
14. Robson SC, Schulte am Esch J, 2nd and Bach FH. Factors in xenograft rejection. *Ann N Y Acad Sci* 1999; 875: 261.
15. Dawson JR, Vidal AC and Malyguine AM. Natural killer cell-endothelial cell interactions in xenotransplantation. *Immunol Res*, 2000; 22(2–3): 165.
16. Pietra BA and Gill RG. Immunobiology of cardiac allograft and xenograft transplantation. *Semin Thorac Cardiovasc Surg Pediatr Card Surg Annu* 2001; 4: 123.
17. Schulte am Esch J, 2nd, Rogiers X and Robson SC. Molecular incompatibilities in hemostasis between swine and men—impact on xenografting. *Ann Transplant* 2001; 6(3): 12.
18. Rose AG. Understanding the pathogenesis and the pathology of hyperacute cardiac rejection. *Cardiovasc Pathol* 2002; 11(3): 171.
19. Ochsenbein AF and Zinkernagel RM. Natural antibodies and complement link innate and acquired immunity. *Immunol Today* 2000; 21(12): 624.
20. Schuurman HJ *et al.* Incidence of hyperacute rejection in pig-to-primate transplantation using organs from hDAF-transgenic donors. *Transplantation* 2002; 73(7): 1146.
21. Dorling A. Are anti-endothelial cell antibodies a prerequisite for the acute vascular rejection of xenografts? *Xenotransplantation* 2003; 10(1): 16.
22. Soares MP *et al.* Accommodation. *Immunol Today* 1999; 20(10): 434.
23. Katori M, Busuttil RW and Kupiec-Weglinski JW. Heme oxygenase-1 system in organ transplantation. *Transplantation* 2002; 74(7): 905.
24. Galili U. Significance of anti-Gal IgG in chronic xenograft rejection. *Transplant Proc* 1999; 31(1–2): 940.
25. Costa C *et al.* Delayed rejection of porcine cartilage is averted by transgenic expression of alpha1,2-fucosyltransferase. *Faseb J* 2003; 17(1): 109.
26. Wallgren AC, Karlsson-Parra A and Korsgren O. The main infiltrating cell in xenograft rejection is a CD4+ macrophage and not a T lymphocyte. *Transplantation* 1995; 60(6): 594.
27. Mohr M *et al.* Recognition of xenogeneic erythrocytes: the GalNAc/Gal-particle receptor of rat liver macrophages mediates or participates in recognition. *Biol Cell* 1987; 60(3): 217.
28. Yamamoto F and Yamamoto M. Molecular genetic basis of porcine histo-blood group AO system. *Blood* 2001; 97(10): 3308.
29. Lewin GA. Repair of a full thickness corneoscleral defect in a German shepherd dog using porcine small intestinal submucosa. *J Small Anim Pract* 1999; 40(7): 340.
30. Ohno K *et al.* Transplantation of cryopreserved human corneas in a xenograft model. *Cryobiology* 2002; 44(2): p. 142.
31. Larkin DF *et al.* Experimental orthotopic corneal xenotransplantation in the rat: mechanisms of graft rejection. *Transplantation* 1995; 60(5): 491.
32. Larkin DF and Williams KA. The host response in experimental corneal xenotransplantation. *Eye* 1995; 9(Pt 2): p. 254.
33. Grueterich M and Tseng SC. Human limbal progenitor cells expanded on intact amniotic membrane *ex vivo*. *Arch Ophthalmol* 2002; 120(6): 783.
34. Bahn CF *et al.* Complications associated with bovine corneal endothelial cell-lined homografts in the cat. *Invest Ophthalmol Vis Sci* 1982; 22(1): 73.

35. Kubo M *et al.* Immunogenicity of human amniotic membrane in experimental xenotransplantation. *Invest Ophthalmol Vis Sci* 2001; 42(7): 1539.
36. Moore MB *et al.* Fate of lyophilized xenogeneic corneal lenticules in intrastromal implantation and epikeratophakia. *Invest Ophthalmol Vis Sci* 1987; 28(3): 555.
37. Tanaka K and Streilein JW. Immunobiology of xenogeneic cornea grafts in mouse eyes: II. Immunogenicity of xenogeneic cornea tissue grafts implanted in anterior chamber of mouse eyes. *Transplantation* 2000; 69(4): 616.
38. Lin Y, Vandeputte M and Waer M. Natural killer cell- and macrophage-mediated rejection of concordant xenografts in the absence of T and B cell responses. *J Immunol* 1997; 158(12): 5658.
39. Kroshus TJ, Bolman RM, 3rd, and Dalmasso AP. Selective IgM depletion prolongs organ survival in an *ex vivo* model of pig-to-human xenotransplantation. *Transplantation* 1996; 62(1): 5.
40. Candinas D *et al.* T cell independence of macrophage and natural killer cell infiltration, cytokine production, and endothelial activation during delayed xenograft rejection. *Transplantation* 1996; 62(12): 1920.
41. Schaapherder AF *et al.* Antibody-dependent cell-mediated cytotoxicity against porcine endothelium induced by a majority of human sera. *Transplantation* 1994; 57(9): 1376.
42. Ross JR, Howell DN and Sanfilippo FP. Characteristics of corneal xenograft rejection in a discordant species combination. *Invest Ophthalmol Vis Sci* 1993; 34(8): 2469.
43. Ross JR, Sanfilippo FP and Howell DN. Histopathologic features of rejecting orthotopic corneal xenografts. *Curr Eye Res* 1994; 13(10): 725.
44. Takano T and Williams KA. Mechanism of corneal endothelial destruction in rejecting rat corneal allografts and xenografts: a role for CD4+ cells. *Transplant Proc* 1995; 27(1): 260.
45. Tanaka K, Yamada J and Streilein JW. Xenoreactive CD4+ T cells and acute rejection of orthotopic guinea pig corneas in mice. *Invest Ophthalmol Vis Sci* 2000; 41(7): 1827.
46. Higuchi R and Streilein JW. CD8+ T cell-mediated delayed rejection of orthotopic guinea pig cornea grafts in mice deficient in CD4+ T cells. *Invest Ophthalmol Vis Sci* 2003; 44(1): 175.
47. Benelli U *et al.* FK-506 delays corneal graft rejection in a model of corneal xenotransplantation. *J Ocul Pharmacol Ther* 1996; 12(4): 425.
48. Liversidge J, Thomson AW and Forrester JV. FK 506 modulates accessory cell adhesion molecule expression and inhibits CD4 lymphocyte adhesion to retinal pigment epithelial cells in vitro: implications for therapy of uveoretinitis. *Transplant Proc* 1991; 23(6): 3339.
49. Tanaka K, Sonoda K and Streilein JW. Acute rejection of orthotopic corneal xenografts in mice depends on CD4(+) T cells and self-antigen-presenting cells. *Invest Ophthalmol Vis Sci* 2001; 42(12): 2878.
50. Liu Y *et al.* Draining lymph nodes of corneal transplant hosts exhibit evidence for donor major histocompatibility complex (MHC) class II-positive dendritic cells derived from MHC class II-negative grafts. *J Exp Med* 2002; 195(2): 259.
51. Hrdličková-Cela E *et al.* Cells of porcine epidermis and corneal epithelium are not recognized by human natural anti-alpha-galactoside IgG. *Folia Biol (Praha)* 2001; 47(6): 200.
52. Goslings WR *et al.* A small molecular weight factor in aqueous humor acts on C1q to prevent antibody-dependent complement activation. *Invest Ophthalmol Vis Sci* 1998; 39(6): 989.

53. Suzuki K *et al.* Cell-matrix and cell-cell interactions during corneal epithelial wound healing. *Prog Retin Eye Res* 2003; 22(2): 113.
54. Bansal, AK and Veenashree MP. Laser refractive surgery: technological advance and tissue response. *Biosci Rep* 2001; 21(4): 491.
55. Wilson SE *et al.* The corneal wound healing response: cytokine-mediated interaction of the epithelium, stroma, and inflammatory cells. *Prog Retin Eye Res* 2001; 20(5): 625.
56. Ohno K *et al.* Keratocyte activation and apoptosis in transplanted human corneas in a xenograft model. *Invest Ophthalmol Vis Sci* 2002; 43(4): 1025.
57. Li C *et al.* Experimental studies on penetrating heterokeratoplasty with human corneal grafts in monkey eyes. *Cornea* 1992; 11(1): 66.
58. Machaty Z *et al.* The use of nuclear transfer to produce transgenic pigs. *Cloning Stem Cells* 2002; 4(1): 21.

8

Animal Models of Corneal Graft

Introduction—Historical Note

The use of animals for penetrating keratoplasty has a long history (see Chapter 1). Since the first attempt at corneal grafting in a domesticated gazelle [1], the value of animal models for the study of the pathogenesis of graft rejection and of potential therapeutic modalities, has been recognized. Even prior to this time there had been some early attempts at corneal grafting in rabbits and chickens by an active school of German ophthalmologists (see [2] for an early review of this period). Most work that has been performed in the rabbit has focussed on investigating not only immunological rejection but also several other phenomena that are seen in humans in failed corneal grafts such as ocular surface disease and retrocorneal membranes [3]. Several reasons underlie the widespread use of the rabbit model including factors such as size of the eye and thus greater similarity to the human graft. However, there are also a number of drawbacks to the rabbit model (see below) and thus later models using small rodents were introduced [4, 5]. These are now the standard of practice for immunological studies while the larger animal models are reserved for modelling human graft rejection and evaluation of clinical signs [6, 7].

Value of Animal Models

The main purpose of animal models of corneal graft is to investigate the pathogenesis and treatment of graft rejection. There are many aspects to the pathogenesis of corneal graft rejection which require careful modelling in the context of human grafts. Corneal grafts in humans are normally performed without tissue or HLA typing as "outbred" grafts, yet still enjoy a high level of acceptance in the first year after grafting [8]. Initial animal models in the rabbit and cat followed these conditions for grafting and produced data which was comparable to the human situation. However, rabbit and cat corneal graft rejection rates are different from the human depending on the type of graft (see below), thus showing that species differences have a significant influence on graft acceptance. The more recent model in the sheep [6] has permitted further analysis of the outbred model and should allow closer correlation of immunological and clinical parameters since there is a wider range of immunological reagents available for the sheep than the rabbit.

The introduction of the rat [4] and more importantly the mouse [5] models of corneal graft rejection has opened up the possibility for more incisive immunological studies. This is due to the extensive knowledge of mouse and rat genetics and the availability of congenic and inbred strains particularly of mice. In addition, there is an increasingly large range of genetically manipulated mice, including transgenic, gene-deleted and conditionally gene-deleted mice. It is now possible to ask specific molecular questions in investigation of the immune response to corneal allografts and xenografts (see Chapters 6 and 7).

From the clinical point of view the mouse and the rat models display significant differences from human grafts for simple anatomical reasons, and in addition the technical expertise required is such that there is greater possibility of surgical trauma with a heightened innate immune response (see Chapter 6 and also below). Despite this, these models, especially the mouse, have led to a much greater understanding of the process of immunological rejection generally and information from this model has revealed the importance of indirect allorecognition generally to the transplantation biologist.

Types of Animal Model

Animal models of corneal graft rejection can be classified into two broad groups: large outbred animal models and small (usually rodent) inbred animal models. The use of these models is determined by the experimental aims. Thus if the aims of the study are to investigate clinical changes to the endothelium by slit lamp biomicroscopy or confocal ophthalmoscopy, the rabbit, cat and sheep have proved valuable and shown similar changes during the graft rejection process to that in the human. However, if the aims of the study are to investigate immunological processes the mouse particularly has been valuable.

With both types of model a significant advantage is the possibility of studying changes in the model from the earliest time after grafting and before the onset of graft rejection, which is not possible in the human.

The rabbit

The rabbit was the first animal model to be used in any planned systematic way for investigation of changes either in the graft or in the secondary lymphoid tissue [9]. Successful corneal grafts in rabbits were reported as long ago as 1930 [10, 11] and several reviews of the procedures have appeared in the literature from time to time [12, 13]. Different models have been used including penetrating keratoplasty (PK), lamellar grafting [14], limbal epithelial grafts [15], and limbal stem cell grafts [16, 17].

In the rabbit, a high rate of successful keratoplasty depends significantly on the size of the graft and the degree of prior corneal vascularization [18] while additional sensitization, e.g. via a later skin graft, further endangers the viability of the graft [19]. Grafts of 7.0 mm in diameter have been reported to reject almost universally in the experience of some authors [9]; in this regard, the rabbit has been hindered to some extent by the rapid and extensive clotting of the aqueous which takes place immediately on entering the anterior chamber and it is possible that this may have had an influence on the outcome. However, this may be a common occurrence in all species but is generally underrecognized. In contrast, smaller grafts of 4–5 mm diameter remain clear indefinitely [19] and it has proved difficult to induce rejection of these grafts. In a well-planned series of experiments, Khodadoust showed that small centrally placed grafts have an excellent survival rate, but similar-sized grafts placed eccentrically and closer to the limbus rejected more readily, particularly when they induced vascularization [19]. It was this work that has highlighted the importance of vascularization of the host graft as a determinant of acceptance but it may require a modified interpretation (see below). Lamellar grafts had a better prognosis than penetrating grafts but both tended to reject in the presence of blood vessels, e.g. when sutures were left in place long enough to cause vascularization. Similar experience has been obtained by others in that prior vascularization in the host graft is required to induce rejection [20]. Prevention of the fibrin response in the anterior chamber, which may last for several days, has been a factor in improving the success rate of rabbit allografts and the use of topical heparin to control this has been important [9]. Despite this, synechiae are a common complication (up to 35% in one study [9]).

Considerable attention to surgical technique is required to avoid wound leakage and cataract formation. Khodadhost improved his technically successful grafts to 95% for 7.0 mm grafts and 100% for 5.0 mm grafts by paying great attention to surgical technique and also by using topical heparin during the procedure to prevent clotting [10]. As with many models, "technical failures" or grafts that fail to clear during the first few days of surgery are usually excluded from analysis. Both interrupted and continuous sutures have been used [21] usually of varying size, initially from 8/0 vicryl to current use of 10/0 nylon. In general, sutures if left in place for longer than 9–10 days induced vascularization crossing the host–graft junction.

The tendency for vessels to be associated with rejection has led to the view that the avascular graft remains clear due to blockade of the efferent arm of the immune response [19]. However, recent studies showing that corneal vascularization is associated with lymphangiogenesis as well as vasculogenesis has promoted the view that increased afferent cell traffic to the draining lymph node might also be a factor in promoting rejection of such grafts [22].

The clinical signs of rejection in the rabbit are a loss of clarity of the donor graft. Rejection is evidenced by initial vascularization followed by opacification of the cornea usually commencing in the vicinity of the new vessels. Since the cornea, unlike the skin, has readily identifiable biomicroscopic *in vivo* components (epithelial, stromal and endothelial layers), an early area for investigation has been to determine which corneal layer induces the strongest alloresponse. A series of elegant experiments, involving the double exchange of corneal grafts between pairs of rabbits which had selective removal of one or more layers of the cornea, thus permitting regrafting of donor–host chimeric grafts to the original donor, has shown that rejection of each of the different layers of the cornea takes place at its own tempo with the epithelium being the first layer to be rejected [23] possibly due to its greater upregulation of MHC Class I after transplantation (see below, and Chapter 6). In this regard, certain signs of rejection do follow the human pattern such as the epithelial and endothelial rejection lines. The epithelial rejection line appears to sweep in advance of the source of vascularization particularly if this is asymmetric or starts predominantly in one sector of the cornea. Histological examination reveals that the line is formed by infiltrating leukocytes beyond which are an advancing field of dead and dying donor epithelial cells. Bringing up the rear is a thin one-to-two-cell-thick layer of host epithelial cells which eventually cover the entire cornea as the rejection line sweeps across the surface. If vascularization is circumferential and uniform, then the rejection line forms a circle which progresses in decreasing radius towards the centre of the cornea and disappears. Donor epithelial replacement is complete by this process in a few weeks. Similar signs can be seen in human corneal graft rejection (see Chapter 3).

A similar endothelial rejection line occurs which is also demarcated by a line of inflammatory, predominantly mononuclear cells migrating behind a retreating sheet of dying endothelial cells. Behind this the endothelial monolayer is either not replaced by cells, or is covered by scattered inflammatory cells and a developing sheet of spindle shaped fibroblastoid cells, eventually going on to form a retrocorneal membrane. In vivo studies of "nonrejecting" rabbit corneal grafts using slit lamp biomicroscopy and confocal ophthalmoscopy have, in some animals, revealed patchy areas of endothelial cell damage [24, 25], previously observed to resemble "pock marks" [26]. Consequently, attempts to investigate the mechanism of this process have used intracameral injection of sensitized lymphocytes which have shown a pattern very similar to the immune process in the rejecting graft [27]. A form of local graft vs host response was suggested which was prescient of the notion later propounded that corneal endothelial cells could induce apoptosis of host lymphocytes via a Fas-FasL-based mechanism and is one of the proposed mechanisms for immune privilege [28] (see Chapter 6).

Overall the rabbit corneal graft has provided useful information over many years but due to the rapid, acute inflammatory response and the lack of a sufficiently wide range of immunological reagents, its value is somewhat limited and its current use has declined significantly.

The cat

Few studies have been performed on the cat as a model of corneal graft. Of those reported the purpose of the studies was to mimic the clinical changes seen in human corneal grafts by a modified form of *in vivo* specular microscopy [7] and by confocal ophthalmoscopy [25]. In one study, attempts were made to evaluate clinically endothelial cell loss due to the alloimmune response. Losses due to the surgery or to prior culture of the donor material were controlled for by using rotational autografts. All donor grafts were cultured in medium for up to 24 hours before grafting.

Graft rejection followed a similar pattern to other large animal models including the human. Essentially, loss of clarity associated with vascularization is a major feature and epithelial and endothelial rejection lines can be observed.

The cat has been a model for determining the usefulness and relevance of endothelial cell counts as a monitor of rejection and graft viability. Endothelial cell loss one month after grafting averaged about 30% of the total donor area. Graft rejection as evidenced by endothelial cell loss in homografts occurred at a level of 15% [7]. In a separate set of experiments in which the endothelium of the donor was removed prior to grafting it was shown that in the cat there was no evidence of regeneration of the endothelium from the host [7].

In a similar experiment endothelial cell counts in corneal homografts declined by nearly 50% in the period between 6 weeks and 9 months following grafting [25]. In addition there was an significant increase in polymegathism. The reasons for this progressive cell loss after homografting was not determined and it could be postulated that it might be due to chronic low level rejection, a little akin to the pock marks seen in the rabbit where small islands of endothelial cells are selectively damaged by alloreactive T cells [26] (see above). However, since there was no correlation with cell loss in corresponding rotational autografts in this study it is difficult to be certain concerning the cause of the endothelial cell loss. This study nevertheless shows the value of using large animal models to mimic the situation in humans since the nature of the endothelial cell loss and the presumed chronic rejection are likely to be similar if for no other reason than through anatomical constraints. Clearly the situation in the rat and mouse is different due to the ocular dimensions and in particular the shallow anterior chamber.

The sheep

The most recent large animal model described for study of corneal graft rejection is the sheep [6] and it is perhaps appropriate that this has been described by a group of Australian researchers. As indicated above, the advantage of using this model is that there is a larger range of immunological reagents to assist study of the cellular and cytokine responses in the cornea than in other large animal models.

The grafting technique described followed a standard pattern: outbred animals of the Morino strain were treated in pairs and a 12 mm diameter trephined graft was transferred between animals. Four cardinal 9/0 ethilon sutures were placed and the graft secured with a continuous suture of the same material. Sutures of narrower bore were found to be insufficiently strong to control the tensions of the healing sheep cornea. No requirement for viscoelastic agents was indicated, nor was heparin used to prevent clotting in the anterior chamber.

Graft rejection was determined using a range of criteria as for the rabbit and the human: the appearance of "rejection lines" signified rejection; in addition, in deference to the rodent grading systems based on oedema and level of corneal opacity, each of these features was graded on a scale of 0–4 with 0 signifying a completely clear (opacity score) and thin (oedema) cornea while 4 represented a totally opaque and maximally thickened cornea as viewed by a hand-held slit lamp (Figure 8.1A, B). Specular microscopy of the endothelium showed the integrity of the monolayer and the value of this model for clinical evaluation of endothelial rejection (Figure 8.2A, B).

As with other models, autografts survived indefinitely although vascularization crossing the graft host junction occurred. However, allografts generally rejected with a mean survival time of only 20 days and in association with considerable vascularization. Fibrin was a constant early feature in allografts and gradually resolved. In addition, keratic precipitates were observed. Clinically rejection was most manifest by spreading oedema and

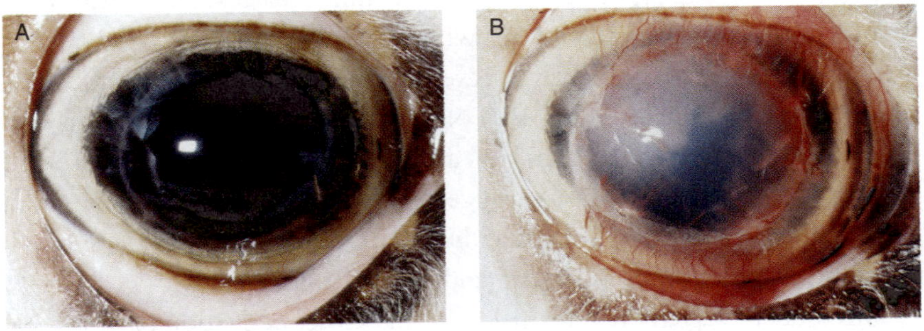

Figure 8.1 Full-thickness penetrating keratoplasty in the sheep. (**A**) Accepted graft; (**B**) rejected graft. (*Courtesy K. Williams.*)

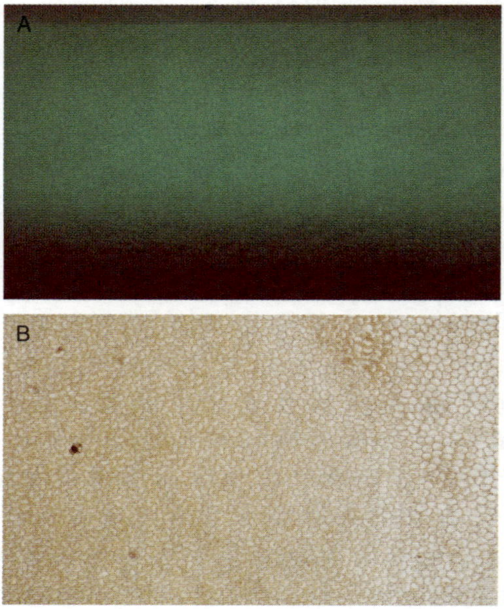

Figure 8.2 Full-thickness penetrating keratoplasty in the sheep. (**A**) Specular microscopy image; (**B**) flat mount preparation. (*Courtesy K. Williams.*)

loss of clarity arising in association with vascularization; other responses similar to those in human such as epithelial and endothelial rejection lines were occasionally observed. Epithelial rejection was associated with upregulation of MHC Class I while endothelial rejection was evidenced by damage or loss of cells. This appeared to be linked to a prominent mononuclear cell response.

Immunohistology of rejected sheep corneal graft showed that the early inflammatory response comprised macrophages and interstitial dendritic cells. CD4+ T cells appeared in the graft within 2 days, which corresponds with studies in the mouse and rat, while CD8+ T cells appeared later by 8 days. Cytokine mRNA analysis revealed the expected raft of proinflammatory molecules including IL-2, TNF-α and INF-γ in allografts. In contrast, the inflammatory response in autografts was signatured with IL-2, TNF-α and IL-10. These results suggest cytokine regulation of the immune versus the tolerant response coinciding with data from other systems in which IL-10 is linked to tolerance and IFN-γ to immunity.

This model thus has the potential to permit closer evaluation of the human corneal graft immune response in which such changes as leukocyte–endothelial cell interactions could be evaluated using methods such as *in vivo* specular microscopy, confocal three- and four-colour microscopy and laser capture microdissection. The model has already been used to evaluate novel treatments including gene therapy (see Chapter 10).

The rat

Penetrating keratoplasty in the rat was first described by Williams *et al.* in 1985 [4]. This was a significant advance in the field since it opened up possibilities for extensive immunological investigation using inbred rat strains and the many rat immunoreagents. Grafts were performed in syngeneic and allogeneic combination usually of fully mismatched MHC antigens and of minor antigens. The standard procedure in the rat eye was to suture a 2.5–3.0 mm donor button into a 2.0–2.5 host bed using 10/0 or 11/0 interrupted sutures. Isografts (Fischer into Fischer) remained clear indefinitely while allografts (DA into Fischer) underwent opacification usually around a mean time of 12 days. Remarkably, in the original study by Williams *et al.* 43% of opacified grafts cleared spontaneously while the remaining grafts remained cloudy and were considered irreversibly rejected.

Several other groups have used the rat corneal allograft model and in most strain combinations, graft rejection has been irreversible [29–32]. In fact the definition of rejection has varied somewhat between studies with some workers taking opacification between 15–25 days as the point of clinical rejection. In the rat this may be acceptable since most strain combinations appear not go through a period transient opacification. However, it makes comparisons of data between studies difficult (see further discussion of this issue below).

Signs of graft rejection in the rat also included several other features including vascularization, corneal oedema and thickening, and patchy infiltration of the stroma presumably by inflammatory cell aggregates. In many studies these were included in an aggregate score but as discussed below for the mouse, corneal opacity is the major clinical determinant of rejection. Rejection lines as seen in larger animal models are not a reliable feature in rat allografts.

The rat PK model has been extremely valuable in permitting studies of cellular mechanisms of graft rejection and of newer approaches to treatment including various monoclonal antibody therapies and potentially gene therapy (see Chapter 10).

The rat has also been valuable for other studies with clinical relevance. Thus "high risk" models of graft rejection have been developed [4] using prior vascularization of the host bed. Interestingly, even in this model some animals underwent spontaneous clearance although the incidence was lower that in allografts into clear corneas.

In addition, models aimed at controlling surface disease using limbal grafts and lamellar grafts have also been utilized [33].

Mouse grafts

The mouse corneal graft model has emerged in recent years as the paradigm for studies of immunological allorejection. Heterotopic mouse corneal grafts in which donor corneas were placed in subcutaneous pockets were described by Chandler *et al.* [34] but orthotopic murine corneal grafts were initially described by She *et al.* [5], since when the model has been taken up by several research groups [5, 35–42] and knowledge of immune mechanisms has advanced through the use of genetically manipulated mice and novel immunologics (see Chapters 6 and 10). Most models are based on the use of a 2.0 mm donor graft placed into a 1.5 or 1.75 mm host bed, secured with 8–12 sutures. More recently, continuous sutures have been used [43, 44] and found to induce less inflammation since they are not removed.

Corneal grafts in the mouse have helped to define clearly the relative roles of direct versus indirect allorecognition (see Chapter 6) but some confusion in the literature has developed concerning the definition of clinical graft rejection. Rejection in the mouse is characterized as for all other species by opacity of the cornea but the several other features identified in the rat are also evident during this process: these include vascularization, infiltration by inflammatory cells, oedema and thickening of the cornea. Grading systems in which aggregate scores of all of these features have been compared to scores using opacity level only have shown that the estimation of the level of opacity provides a sufficiently reliable measure of clinical rejection (for review see [44]) (Figures 8.3A–E).

However, opacity of the cornea in itself may be insufficient to signify irreversible rejection (see discussion below). As in the rat, transient opacification of the cornea, several days after allografting, has been observed frequently and appears to relate to the degree of surgical trauma since it occurs only when interrupted sutures are used to secure the graft and usually shortly after the sutures are removed. In contrast, continuous sutures are not usually associated with transient opacification although the eventual rejection rate for both interrupted and continuous sutures is similar. Thus

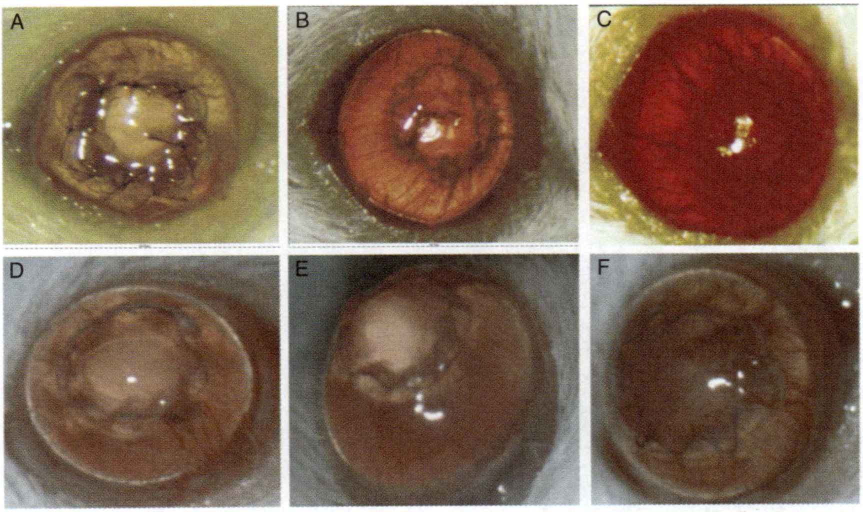

Figure 8.3 Full-thickness penetrating keratoplasty in the mouse. (**A**) Clear graft, interrupted suture; (**B**) clear graft, sutures removed; (**C**) rejected graft; (**D**) clear graft, continuous suture; (**E**) clear graft, oblique view; (**F**) rejected graft, continuous suture.

both opacity level and persistence of opacification are probably essential criteria of irreversible rejection in the mouse (see below) while reduced opacity alone is sufficient to signify, although not pathognomic of, a rejection episode.

Studies in the mouse have provided a flood information on the immunological mechanisms of graft rejection (see Chapter 6). Thus long lasting controversies for instance regarding the role of MHC antigens, the need for tissue typing and matching, the role of indirect rather that direct mechanism, CD4+ T cells rather than CD8 cytotoxic cells, antigen presentation and costimulation by host and donor cells, roles of antibody, cytokines and chemokines have all been addressed and are constantly being refined. In addition, avenues are now open to investigate many possible new therapeutic strategies (see Chapter 10).

However, the mouse also has its limitations. In particular, it is difficult to correlate precisely the clinical features of mouse graft rejection and human graft rejection. In addition, that interesting period when the cornea is under immunological attack but not yet irreversibly damaged (i.e. the rejection episode) is the point of greatest clinical relevance to the practicing clinician and may not be adequately modelled in small animal such as the rat and the mouse.

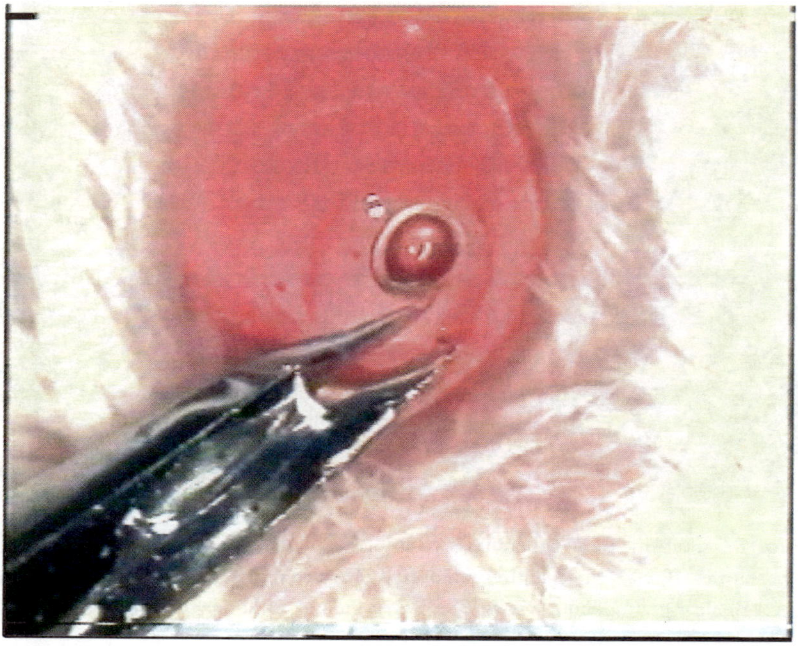

Figure 8.4 Preparation of host cornea bed for full-thickness penetrating keratoplasty in the mouse (see also video clips on CD).

Despite these caveats, the immunologist has much to gain from the mouse model since it represents a model of solid organ transplant rejection which is almost exclusively underwritten by indirect allorecognition and chronic rejection which are now increasingly recognized as major components of graft rejection generally. For this work, the mouse corneal allograft model is a useful system provided mastery of the surgical technique is not found to be too much of a deterrent (Figure 8.4 plus CD movie).

Clinical Criteria of Graft Rejection

Rejection in solid tissue allografts is determined by a range of tests, including clinical (e.g. cardiac), biochemical/metabolic (e.g. renal and pancreatic), and often finally by pathological examination of the rejected graft. Thus criteria for rejection vary with the tissue and may not be comparable between tissues. This applies particularly to the skin and cornea: rejection of skin grafts is a clear end stage event visualized by discoloration and sloughing of the tissue. In contrast, rejection of the cornea is characterized principally by loss of clarity (opacification) of the tissue but the tissue is not usually sloughed unless in the case of small xenografts. In addition, opacification of the cornea can be reversible: in humans early signs of epithelial oedema and inflammatory cell deposits on the endothelium can disappear if the eye is treated sufficiently with appropriate immunosuppressive therapy. In this case it is frequently called a "rejection episode". However, when sufficiently advanced the development of epithelial and even more so of endothelial rejection lines is a poor prognostic indicator for the survival of the graft.

In experimental animals, similar rejection episodes occur. However, in large animal models, and especially if untreated, evidence of rejection lines associated with vascularization is a harbinger of an inexorable process leading to the eventual total rejection of the graft. In the sheep, this results in a totally scleralized, opaque white cornea (Williams, personal communication) in 100% of cases. (Figure 8.1B). In rabbits, cats and sheep, this may reflect the fact that these grafts are performed in outbred, presumably fully mismatched animals.

In the rat and mouse transient opacification of the cornea can occur. According to the criteria for clinical graft rejection, this transient opacification can be severe enough to signify total rejection (i.e. an opacity score greater that two [38] yet the cornea can become transparent again after a period of several days or weeks. There has been considerable controversy over the nature of this phenomenon seen in rat and mouse grafts. Corneal clarity is maintained predominantly by a healthy endothelium which pumps fluid out of the cornea into the aqueous humour. In larger animals in which endothelial cell loss could be observed by specular or confocal microscopy, (Figure 8.2A), opacification of the cornea was indeed associated with endothelial cell loss, usually without recovery [7, 25, 45], and in some cases replacement by a fibroblastic retrocorneal membrane. In the rat and mouse, therefore, transient opacification of the graft was considered to be due to loss of donor endothelium, and it was assumed that later clearing of the graft represented proliferation of the host endothelium to cover the donor button. This was based on experiments showing that the corneal endothelium in certain species such as the rabbit and the rat has the potential to proliferate after injury [46–48]. However, there is no evidence that the host endothelium can re-cover a donor corneal allograft, and even on an isograft removal of the endothelium before graft emplacement is not reliably followed by host endothelial cell proliferation to cover the graft [49]. This may partly be due to the fact that a denuded corneal stroma (Descemet's membrane) is an unsuitable surface for growth of normally poorly dividing host endothelial cells. It is also possible that a continuing macrophage-rich alloimmune response which is present on rejected corneal donor grafts also is a poor environment for a reparative host endothelial cell response.

How is it possible therefore to explain the recovery of clarity by mouse and rat corneal grafts that have apparently been clinically "rejected"? Experiments involving allogeneic C57Bl6 corneas from the Green Fluorescent Protein (GFP)-transgenic mouse, in which all nucleated cells express GFP and are thus identifiable by immunofluorescent confocal microscopy, were transplanted to normal Balb/c mice have shown that rejected opaque grafts evaluated after 56 days, had lost all donor endothelium. In contrast, clear grafts some of which must have passed through a period of transient "rejection" between 10 and 21 days, retained donor endothelium. In similar experiments (Plšková, Kuffová and Forrester, in progress), attempts were made to correlate corneal opacity level with percentage viability of the corneal endothelium. It was found that on average, a minimal level of corneal endothelial cell coverage (>48%) was required to maintain a clinically nonrejected clear cornea (opacity level 1.0 or less) but that the correlation was not perfect. In fact, some corneas with greater that 90% endothelial cell coverage displayed a level of opacity up to 4.0 (strong evidence of rejection [38]), while other corneas with almost totally absent endothelium had opacity levels <2.0.

Thus the most reliable criterion of irreversible corneal allograft rejection in the experimental model is evaluation of the integrity of the endothelial monolayer. In large animal models this can be done by specular microscopy (Figure 8.2A) and confocal ophthalmoscopy, in rats and mice histopathological examination of flat mounts of the cornea is the method of choice. Clinically a combination of corneal opacity level greater that 2.0, persisting for a period of 56 days, would be required to categorize any cornea as irreversibly rejected. This has been previously suggested empirically [38] on the basis of extensive experimental experience in mice and fits with the notion that corneal allograft rejection as a model of indirect allorecognition represents chronic rather than acute rejection.

Conclusion

A range of animal models is available to study immunological and functional changes that occur during corneal graft rejection. Different models offer different advantages for specific studies. In designing studies with clear aims, it is valuable to ensure that the model used provides an endpoint which reflects the question under study.

References

1. Bigger SI. Inquiry into the possibility of transplanting the corneas, with the view of relieving blindness (hitherto deemed uncurable) caused by several diseases of that structure. *Dublin J Med Sci* 1837; 11: 408.
2. Rycroft B. The corneal graft—past, present and future. *Trans Ophthalmol Soc UK* 1965; 85: 459.
3. Rycroft PV. Corneal graft membranes. *Trans Ophthalmol Soc UK* 1965; 85: p. 317.
4. Williams KA and Coster DJ. Penetrating corneal transplantation in the inbred rat: a new model. *Invest Ophthalmol Vis Sci* 1985; 26(1): 23.
5. She SC, Steahly LP and Moticka EJ. A method for performing full-thickness, orthotopic, penetrating keratoplasty in the mouse. *Ophthalmic Surg* 1990; 21(11): 781.
6. Williams KA. *et al.* A new model of orthotopic penetrating corneal transplantation in the sheep: graft survival, phenotypes of graft-infiltrating cells and local cytokine production. *Aust N Z J Ophthalmol* 1999; 27(2): 127.
7. Cohen KL. *et al.* Cat endothelial morphology after corneal transplant. *Curr Eye Res* 1990; 9(5): 445.
8. The collaborative corneal transplantation studies (CCTS): Effectiveness of histocompatibility matching in high-risk corneal transplantation. The Collaborative Corneal Transplantation Studies Research Group. *Arch Ophthalmol* 1992; 110(10): 1392.
9. Bourne WM *et al.* The effect of splenectomy on corneal graft rejection. *Invest Ophthalmol* 1976; 15(7): 541
10. Khodadoust AA. Penetrating keratoplasty in the rabbit. *Am J Ophthalmol* 1968; 66(5): 899.
11. Thomas JWT. Transplantation of the cornea: a preliminary report on a series of experiments on rabbits, together with a demonstration of four rabbits with clear corneal grafts. *Trans Ophthalmol Soc UK* 1930; 50: 127.
12. Castroviejo R. Keratoplasty: an historical and experimental study, including a new method: part II. *Am J Ophthalmol* 1932; 15: 905.
13. Stansbury FC and Wadsworth JAC. Surgical technique of corneal transplantation in rabbits. *Am J Ophthalmol* 1947; 30: 968.
14. Khodadoust AA. Lamellar corneal transplant in the rabbit. *Am J Ophthalmol* 1968; 66: 1111.
15. Tseng SC and Tsai RJ. Limbal transplantation for ocular surface reconstruction—a review. *Fortschr Ophthalmol* 1991; 88(3): 236.
16. Swift GJ *et al.* Survival of rabbit limbal stem cell allografts. *Transplantation* 1996; 62(5): 568.
17. Li QJ *et al.* Long-term survival of allogeneic donor cell-derived corneal epithelium in limbal deficient rabbits. *Curr Eye Res* 2001; 23(5): 336.

18. Hill JC and Maske R. An animal model for corneal graft rejection in high-risk keratoplasty. *Transplantation* 1988; 46(1): 26.
19. Khodadoust AA and Silverstein AM. Studies on the nature of the privilege enjoyed by corneal allografts. *Invest Ophthalmol* 1972; 11(3): 137.
20. Williams KA *et al.* A comparison of the effects of topical cyclosporine and topical steroid on rabbit corneal allograft rejection. *Transplantation* 1985; 39(3): 242.
21. Eliason JA and McCulley JP. A comparison between interrupted and continuous suturing techniques in keratoplasty. *Cornea* 1990; 9(1): 10.
22. Mimura T *et al.* Expression of vascular endothelial growth factor C and vascular endothelial growth factor receptor 3 in corneal lymphangiogenesis. *Exp Eye Res* 2001; 72(1): 71.
23. Khodadoust AA and Silverstein AM. Transplantation and rejection of individual cell layers of the cornea. *Invest Ophthalmol* 1969; 8(2): 180.
24. Cho BJ *et al.* In vivo confocal microscopic analysis of corneal allograft rejection in rabbits. *Cornea* 1998. 17(4): 417.
25. Cohen RA *et al.* Confocal microscopy of corneal graft rejection. *Cornea* 1995; 14(5): 467.
26. Khodadoust AA and Silverstein AM. Local graft versus host reactions within the anterior chamber of the eye: the formation of corneal endothelial pocks. *Invest Ophthalmol* 1975; 14(9): 640.
27. Khodadoust AA and Silverstein AM. Induction of corneal graft rejection by passive cell transfer. *Invest Ophthalmol* 1976; 15(2): 89.
28. Griffith TS. *et al.* Fas ligand-induced apoptosis as a mechanism of immune privilege. *Science* 1995; 270(5239): 1189.
29. Callanan DG *et al.* Histopathology of rejected orthotopic corneal grafts in the rat. *Invest Ophthalmol Vis Sci* 1989; 30(3): 413.
30. He YG. *et al.* Acceptance of H-Y-disparate corneal grafts despite concomitant immunization of the recipient. *Transplantation* 1991; 51(6): 1258.
31. Larkin DF, Calder VL and Lightman SL. Identification and characterization of cells infiltrating the graft and aqueous humour in rat corneal allograft rejection. *Clin Exp Immunol,* 1997; 107(2): 381.
32. Tchah H, Youn DH and Holland EJ. Experimental orthotopic penetrating keratoplasty—a rat penetrating keratoplasty model. *J Korean Med Sci* 1991; 6(1): 15.
33. Amano S, Sawa M and Ishii Y. Keratoepithelioplasty in rat: development of a model and histological study. *Jpn J Ophthalmol* 1992; 36(4): 407.
34. Chandler JW, Ray-Keil L and Gillette TE. Experimental corneal allograft rejection: description of murine model and a new hypothesis of immunopathogenesis. *Curr Eye Res* 1982; 2(6): 387.
35. Lau CH, Nicholls SM and Easty DL. A murine model of interlamellar corneal transplantation. *Br J Ophthalmol* 1998; 82(3): 294.
36. Zhang EP, Schrunder S and Hoffmann F. Orthotopic corneal transplantation in the mouse—a new surgical technique with minimal endothelial cell loss. *Graefes Arch Clin Exp Ophthalmol* 1996; 234(11): 714.
37. He YG, Ross J and Niederkorn JY. Promotion of murine orthotopic corneal allograft survival by systemic administration of anti-CD4 monoclonal antibody. *Invest Ophthalmol Vis Sci* 1991; 32(10): 2723.

38. Sonoda Y and Streilein JW. Orthotopic corneal transplantation in mice—evidence that the immunogenetic rules of rejection do not apply. *Transplantation* 1992; 54(4): 694.
39. Joo CK, Pepose JS and Stuart PM. T-cell mediated responses in a murine model of orthotopic corneal transplantation. *Invest Ophthalmol Vis Sci* 1995; 36(8): 1530.
40. Hašková Z, Filipec M and Holáň V. The role of major and minor histocompatibility antigens in orthotopic corneal transplantation in mice. *Folia Biol (Praha)* 1996; 42(3): 105.
41. Yamagami S and Tsuru T. Increase in orthotopic murine corneal transplantation rejection rate with anterior synechiae. *Invest Ophthalmol Vis Sci* 1999; 40(10): 2422.
42. Hori J and Streilein J W. Dynamics of donor cell persistence and recipient cell replacement in orthotopic corneal allografts in mice. *Invest Ophthalmol Vis Sci* 2001; 42(8): 1820.
43. Kuffová L *et al.* Kinetics of leukocyte and myeloid cell traffic in the murine corneal allograft response. *Transplantation* 2001; 72(7): 1292.
44. Plšková J *et al.* Evaluation of corneal graft rejection in a mouse model. *Br J Ophthalmol* 2002; 86(1): 108.
45. Bahn CF *et al.* Penetrating keratoplasty in the cat: a clinically applicable model. *Ophthalmology* 1982; 89(6): 687.
46. Tuft SJ, Williams KA and Coster DJ. Endothelial repair in the rat cornea. *Invest Ophthalmol Vis Sci* 1986; 27(8): 1199.
47. Schubert HD and Trokel S. Endothelial repair following Nd:YAG laser injury. *Invest Ophthalmol Vis Sci* 1984; 25(8): 971.
48. Olsen EG and Davanger M. The healing of rabbit corneal endothelium. *Acta Ophthalmol (Copenh)* 1984; 62(5): 796.
49. Joo CK *et al.* Repopulation of denuded murine Descemet's membrane with life-extended murine corneal endothelial cells as a model for corneal cell transplantation. *Graefes Arch Clin Exp Ophthalmol* 2000; 238(2): 174.

9

Pathology of Human Corneal Transplantation

Introduction

Corneal transplantation-keratoplasty represents the most common and successful solid organ transplantation in humans [1]. Such a high success in uncomplicated cases is attributed to the properties of normal, healthy corneal tissue and to the microenvironment in the anterior segment of the eye, and particularly anterior chamber, of the eye [2]. Unfortunately, in patients with "high risk" characteristics, the major cause of corneal graft failure still remains immune reaction-rejection against the corneal graft (see Chapter 3) [1].

Pathological studies of human corneal graft rejection are few. There are obvious ethical reasons for this lack of information concerning the cells that infiltrate the cornea during acute graft rejection but studies of the chronic or late phase of rejection are also scarce.

Analysis of Paracentesis Samples During Graft Rejection

A small set of experimental and clinical studies of the cellular and protein content of aqueous humour during the acute phase of corneal rejection epizode have been performed [3–7]. CD4+ T cells were present in the early stage of the rejection epizode in greater numbers over CD8+ T cells in aqueous humour of the rats. In the later phase of rejection the ratio of CD4+/CD8+ T cells changed in favour of CD8 cells [3, 4].

In the human form of the acute rejection episode, increased numbers of monocytes and lymphocytes were detected in the aqueous humour, but granulocytes were infrequent [5]. The increased numbers of monocytes and lymphocytes correlated with severity of the rejection episode [5].

In other studies, cytokines in aqueous humour were measured [6, 7]. Dekaris *et al.* [6]. measured the concentration of TGF-β2 in a series of patients with noninflammatory and inflammatory corneal diseases (high vs low risk recipients). In the noninflammatory situation the concentration of TGF-β2 was similar to that of controls, but in inflammatory corneal diseases, the concentration of TGF-β2 in aqueous humour was significantly lower [6]. In the study of van Gelderen *et al.* the levels of total protein and IL-6 were increased in the aqueous humour prior to penetrating keratoplasty in eyes with previous inflammation [7]. Increased intraocular levels of other proinflammatory cytokines such as IFN-γ, but also noninflammatory cytokines such as IL-10 were observed during the acute phase of corneal rejection. Unfortunately, these results could not predict the final clinical outcome of the graft [7].

Immunohistological Studies of Failed Corneal Grafts

MHC antigens

Corneal epithelial and stromal cells express under normal conditions low levels of MHC class I antigens (see Chapter 5) [8, 9] and do not express MHC class II antigens. MHC class II antigens are found only on Langerhans cells (intraepithelial dendritic cells, DC) in normal human conjunctiva and corneal limbal epithelium [8] and in limbal vascular endothelium [10]. In contrast, HLA class II antigens are found widely distributed on many cell types in pathological corneas [11–13]. The frequency of dendritic cells (DC), the main cell subpopulation expressing MHC class II antigens, in a study Philipp *et al.* was similar to that in the normal epidermis in corneas with epidermalization after severe alkali burns [14]. Numerous Langerhans cells and DC, albeit in smaller numbers, were also present in the central corneal epithelium of patients with keratitis due to a variety of causes, including herpes simplex virus, herpes zoster virus, bacterial corneal ulcers, corneal scars, corneal ulcers associated with rheumatoid arthritis, and patients with chronic corneal allograft rejection [14].

An important study by Williams *et al.* revealed significantly more infiltrating cells bearing one or more of the leucocyte-common antigens (CD45RA, RB and RO), HLA class II antigens, various myeloid-lineage markers, and a peripheral T cell marker, in the graft beds of recipients who subsequently lost a corneal graft than in the graft beds of those for whom the outcome was successful [15]. The hypothesis that large numbers of leucocytes in the recipient graft bed would be correlated with subsequent graft failure was examined by clinical corneal graft survival analysis and results showed that recipients whose corneas contained fewer than 50 leucocyte-common antigen-positive cells/mm^2 of corneal stroma showed a 3-year actuarial graft survival of 83%, compared with 39% in those whose corneas contained more than 50 such cells/mm^2 [15].

The presence of DC, HLA class II+ or Leu-6+ (CD1a+) cells were reported also in studies by Pepose *et al.* and Catry *et al.* [16, 17]. These cells were found in the central corneal epithelium in corneas which were previously rejected and were presumed to be conjunctival Langerhans cells which had migrated from the limbal region. In the study by Kuffová *et al.* DC were detected in corneal epithelium and also in the corneal stroma by dual immunohistochemistry staining [18] (see Chapter 6, Figure 6.1). The presence in the corneal stroma of MHC class II+CD1a+CD19– DC in failed, previously rejected corneal grafts indicated a bone marrow origin for these cells and, in view of the short half life of DCs, suggested continued recruitment of DC to the rejected graft. It was also suggested that these cells are responsible for initiating graft rejection as DC are the only cells capable of transporting alloantigen to the secondary lymphoid organs for presentation to allospecific naive T cells (see Chapter 6).

The presence and persistence of DC in diseased corneas may account for, at least in part, a breakdown of corneal immune privilege, with a higher rate of rejection episodes after corneal transplantation. Furthermore, DC as the most potent antigen-presenting cells in the organism, also play an important role in the initiation and the progression of immune responses in various inflammatory corneal diseases.

T cells and macrophages

The central cornea under the normal conditions is devoid of lymphocytes. In contrast, the periphery of the normal human cornea contains a small population of CD4+ T cells [19]. Extensive studies on the composition of infiltrating cells have been conducted on corneas which previously were rejected [16, 20–22]. In the study by Pepose *et al.* most of cellular infiltrate comprised T cells and macrophages [16]. In the study by Larkin *et al.* a high proportion of graft stroma-infiltrating cells expressed leucocyte common antigen. These were mostly T cells or macrophages [20], and some appeared to be engaged in keratocyte killing as evidenced by the close leucocyte–keratocyte apposition, the regional loss of keratocytes and presence of apoptotic keratocytes. Such changes were observed in all corneal graft rejection specimens, but not in nonrejected control grafts. Interestingly, those grafts which were removed earliest following onset of immunological rejection had the densest graft inflammatory infiltrates. A further consistent finding in all rejected corneal grafts was attenuation of the endothelial cell monolayer which correlated with clinically detected endothelial rejection lines and other signs of rejection [20].

T cell specificity, under the surrogate of oligoclonality, from rejected and nonrejected corneas has been examined. In the study by Wackenheim-Urlacher *et al.* a method for the extraction and propagation of T lymphocytes from rejected, normal, and diseased corneas was developed [21]. Corneas with keratoconus or pseudophakic bullous keratopathy failed to generate T cell lines. From normal corneas activated CD8+ T cells with cytotoxic function were cultured but no CD4+ T cell lines. In contrast, CD4+ and CD8+ T cell lines were successfully grown from rejected corneas. The phenotypic repertoire of the cultured cells was studied by FACS analysis. Rejected corneas were invaded by a mixture of activated CD4+ and CD8+ T cells, with one population being predominant. This suggests that not all alloantigens participate in the rejection response to corneal allografts, compared to other solid organ grafts in which there is polyclonal activation of T cells. That only a restriced set of T cell clones are activated during corneal graft rejection confirms the process of indirect allorecognition.

Systemic cellular responses have also been studied. Human peripheral blood mononuclear leucocytes were investigated in the study by Young *et al.* [22]. Samples were collected at intervals prior and after corneal transplantation surgery and during and after a rejection episode. A direct positive correlation between elevation of Leu-2a+ (CD8+ T cells) following an acute immmune rejection and good final outcome of the corneal graft was found.

Adhesion Molecules and Human Corneal Grafts

Leucocyte adhesion molecules are believed to play a critical role in the selective recruitment of different leucocyte populations to inflammatory sites (see Chapter 6). In numerous immunohistochemistry studies the presence of different adhesion molecules were detected in normal and also pathological corneas [23–25]. Intercellular adhesion molecule-1 (ICAM-1) was focally expressed on corneal epithelial cells and its expression was increased on keratocytes, and corneal and vascular endothelial cells particularly at the site of dense infiltration with mononuclear leucocytes [23]. ICAM-1 was detected also in corneas with herpetic stromal keratitis, zoster keratitis, chemical burns, atopic keratitis, fungal keratitis, and bacterial keratitis [24]. E-selectin was present on endothelial cells of vessels in the stroma of rejected corneal allografts which were characterized by dense infiltration with T cells and macrophages. Vascular cell adhesion molecule-1 (VCAM-1) was predominantly expressed on inflammatory cells of the macrophage/monocyte lineage, but only sporadically on vascular endothelial cells in the stroma of vascularized rejected corneal allografts, in corneas with herpetic stromal keratitis, chemical burns, and atopic keratitis [23, 24]. Potentially blockade of adhesion molecules and their ligands with monoclonal antibodies or their inactive ligands may inhibit and/or completely diminish development of corneal graft rejection and corneal inflammation (see Chapter 10).

Conclusion

Information from human immunohistological studies has been informative only to a limited degree. T cells, monocyte/macrophages and dendritic cells are seen as the main players in this process but how they co-ordinate the rejection response in man is not clear. More extensive studies on the composition of the graft infiltrating lymphocytes have been performed in animal models (see Chapter 6). The presence of macrophages as major subpopulation infiltrating corneal graft, but also CD4+, CD8+ T cells and DC parallel findings in human grafts. Moreover, the findings in secondary lymphoid organs (draining lymph nodes) indicate the crucial role of DC as very potent antigen presenting cells, which are the only cells capable of activating naive T cells. It is likely that an early influx of macrophages is a part of early (surgery-induced) innate immune response and a later secondary infiltraton occurs in reponse to the release of various locally produced chemokines and cytokines by alloreactive T cells but also by corneal parenchymal cells. This amplifies the chemoattraction of antigen-specific T cells and macrophages with further tissue damage and finally complete corneal graft failure.

References

1. The collaborative corneal transplantation studies (CCTS): Effectiveness of histocompatibility matching in high-risk corneal transplantation. The Collaborative Corneal Transplantation Studies Research Group. *Arch Ophthalmol* 1992; 110(10): 1392.
2. Stuart PM, Griffith TS, Usui N, Pepose J, Yu X and Ferguson TA. CD95 ligand (FasL)-induced apoptosis is necessary for corneal allograft survival. *J Clin Invest* 1997; 99(3): 396.
3. Larkin DF, Calder VL and Lightman SL. Identification and characterization of cells infiltrating the graft and aqueous humour in rat corneal allograft rejection. *Clin Exp Immunol* 1997; 107(2): 381.
4. Williams KA, Standfield SD, Mills RA, Takano T, Larkin DF, Krishnan R, Russ GR and Coster DJ. A new model of orthotopic penetrating corneal transplantation in the sheep: graft survival, phenotypes of graft-infiltrating cells and local cytokine production. *Aust N Z J Ophthalmol* 1999; 27(2): 127.
5. Reinhard T *et al.* Immune cells in the anterior chamber of patients with immune reactions after penetrating keratoplasty. *Cornea* 2002; 21(1): 56.
6. Dekaris I, Gabric N, Mazuran R, Karaman Z and Mravicic I. Profile of cytokines in aqueous humour from corneal graft recipients. *Croat Med J* 2001;42(6): 650.
7. van Gelderen BE, Van Der Lelij A, Peek R, Broersma L, Treffers WF, Ruijter JM and van der Gaag R. Cytokines in aqueous humour and serum before and after corneal transplantation and during rejection. *Ophthalmic Res* 2000; 32(4): 157.
8. Fujikawa LS, Calvin RB, Bhan AK *et al.* Expression of HLA-A/B/C and -DR locus antigens on epithelial, stromal and endothelial cells of the human cornea. *Cornea* 1982; 1: 213.
9. Whitsett CF and Stulting RD. The distribution of HLA antigens on human corneal tissue. *Invest Ophthalmol Vis Sci* 1984; 25: 519.
10. Pels E and van der Gaag R. HLA-A,B,C and HLA-DR antigens and dedritic cells in fresh and organ culture preserved corneas. *Cornea* 1985; 3: 231.
11. Delbosc B, Fellmann D, Piquot X *et al. Antigenicite HLA des cornees humaines normales et pathologiques. J Fr Ophthalmol* 1990; 11: 535.
12. Williams KA, Ash JK and Coster DJ. Histocompatibility antigen and passenger cell content of normal and diseased human cornea. *Transplantation* 1985; 39(3): 265.
13. Pepose JS, Gardner KM, Nestor MS, Foos RY and Pettit TH. Detection of HLA class I and II antigens in rejected human corneal allografts. *Ophthalmology* 1985; 92(11): 1480.
14. Philipp W and Gottinger W. Incidence and function of Langerhans cells in various corneal diseases. *Fortschr Ophthalmol* 1990; 87(2): 124.
15. Williams KA, White MA, Ash JK and Coster DJ. Leukocytes in the graft bed associated with corneal graft failure: analysis by immunohistology and actuarial graft survival. *Ophthalmology* 1989; 96(1): 38.
16. Pepose JS, Nestor MS, Gardner KM, Foos RY and Pettit TH. Composition of cellular infiltrates in rejected human corneal allografts. *Graefes Arch Clin Exp Ophthalmol* 1985; 222(3): 128.
17. Catry L, van den Oord J, Foets B *et al.* Morphologic and immunophenotypic heterogenity of corneal dendritic cells. *Graefes Arch Clin Exp Ophthalmol* 1991; 229: 182.

18. Kuffová L, Holáň V, Lumsden L, Forrester JV and Filipec M. Cell subpopulations in failed human corneal grafts. *Br J Ophthalmol* 1999; 83(12): 1364.
19. Scheiffarth OF, Stefani FH, Gabriel N and Lund OE. T lymphocytes of the normal human cornea. *Br J Ophthalmol* 1987; 71(5): 384.
20. Larkin DF, Alexander RA and Cree IA. Infiltrating inflammatory cell phenotypes and apoptosis in rejected human corneal allografts. *Eye* 1997; 11(Pt 1): 68.
21. Wackenheim-Urlacher A, Kantelip B, Falkenrodt A, Piqot X, Tongio MM, Montard M and Delbosc B. T-cell repertoire of normal, rejected, and pathological corneas: phenotype and function. *Cornea* 1995; 14(5): 450.
22. Young E and Stark WJ. Immunology of corneal allograft rejection: associated human leukocyte populations. *Ophthalmology* 1985; 92(2): 223.
23. Philipp W. Leukocyte adhesion molecules in rejected corneal allografts. *Graefes Arch Clin Exp Ophthalmol* 1994; 232(2): 87.
24. Philipp W and Gottinger W. Leukocyte adhesion molecules in diseased corneas. *Invest Ophthalmol Vis Sci* 1993; 34(8): 2449.
25. Whitcup SM, Nussenblatt RB, Price FW Jr and Chan CC. Expression of cell adhesion molecules in corneal graft failure. *Cornea* 1993; 12(6): 475.

10

Therapeutic Approach to Experimental Corneal Graft Rejection

Introduction

Corneal grafts in humans, whether "high" or "low risk", are mandatorily treated with topical steroids from the day of grafting. In contrast, experimental corneal grafts are performed for reasons which may or may not demand immediate postoperative cover with topical immunotherapy. Large grafts performed to determine the behaviour of different cell layers by confocal ophthalmoscopy or specular microscopy may be treated as for human corneal grafts, but experimental keratoplasty performed to investigate immunological mechanisms is normally performed to include an untreated control group. The minimum therapy for most procedures is to apply local antibiotics at the finish of surgery to reduce the incidence of infection.

The therapeutic approach to experimental corneal graft rejection therefore depends on the aims of the experiment, the model, and the incidence and timing of graft rejection. For instance, effective immunotherapy for small allografts in the rabbit, which have a high acceptance rate (see Chapter 8) are likely to be ineffective for xenografts in the mouse (see Chapter 7). It is therefore important to compare like with like in any study of graft outcome and this should be simpler to achieve for experimental studies compared to clinical studies. However, in order to compare data from different laboratories agreement must be reached regarding such parameters as the definition of rejection which is different for different models (see Chapter 8). In addition, even within the same model, different groups have applied different criteria of rejection, thus making comparisons difficult. In addition, strain combination differences produce different base-line levels of rejection (compare for instance graft rejection incidence in C57B6 (H-2^b)→Balb/C (H-2^d) mice with the reverse combination). Finally, the conditions for breeding and housing the experimental animal, the surgical technique and the general level of care have a significant bearing on graft outcome through important innate immune mechanisms (see Chapter 6).

Despite these caveats, experimental investigations of corneal graft rejection have produced some important advances in our understanding of disease mechanisms and have led to novel approaches to the management of human corneal graft rejection.

Strategies for Immunotherapy

The experimental approach will depend on the type of graft and the aim of the treatment, e.g. whether directed toward the innate or adaptive immune response, the afferent or the effector stage of rejection.

Types of graft

The main consideration here is whether in the untreated animal model rejection is 100% or whether there is some level of spontaneous graft acceptance. In humans, unmatched allogeneic grafts in "low risk" situations enjoy a high degree of successful acceptance; in outbred, unmatched sheep rejection is 100%; in xenografts in most animal models rejection is 100%; in MHC matched or MHC unmatched mice rejection rates are similar (varying between 50 and 60%, depending on the laboratory), whereas in non-MHC unmatched grafts rejection rates are significantly higher. Defining the experimental conditions prior to the therapeutic trial is clearly important but more important is interpreting and extrapolating data only in the context of similarly designed experiments.

Blocking the immune respsonse

Also important at the outset of the experiment is a clear idea of which aspect of the immune response is to be modulated. For most immunological reagents, there is usually one or more clear hypotheses to be tested, e.g. inhibition of chemokine action, or induction of a Th2 response. However, for some agents, particularly more broadly acting drugs, the mechanisms of action may not be so clear and in fact it is the drug which is being studied and not its effect on graft rejection. In this situation, it is critically important to have defined graft rejection end-points.

Innate immunity

Until recently, the importance of innate immunity in graft rejection was not articulated, although most corneal surgeons recognized the deleterious effects of apparently trivial events such as loosening of sutures as initiators of graft rejection. Now that there is a greater understanding of the immunological mechanisms of this important response, effort directed towards modulating the effects of cells such as NK cells and macrophages is likely to be intensified.

Adaptive immunity

Historically aspects of adaptive immunity have been the focus of attention and the aim here has been to develop antigen specific therapy in the belief that such approaches will avoid the side effects of the more broad spectrum drugs commonly in use. While some aspects are relatively non-antigen-specific, e.g. inhibition of cellular infiltration by blocking adhesion molecules, other approaches have been targeted towards corneal antigens, e.g. oral tolerance induction. Both the afferent and efferent arms of the response have been extensively investigated.

Drug Delivery

Treatment of ocular diseases offers the possibility of novel drug delivery systems. Systemic delivery of anti-inflammatory and immunosuppressant drugs is frequently used to achieve control of ocular and intraocular inflammation but is associated with significant side effects. Topical application of drugs is standard for many conditions. This particularly applies to corneal grafts in which topical application of steroids plays a significant part in modifying the allograft response.

Systemic immunosuppressants are therefore not commonly used to control graft rejection responses either prophylactically or as therapy. Even with "high risk" grafts and alternative immunosuppressants, topical, subconjunctival and periocular application of drugs are frequently preferred. In addition, different drug vehicles are available such as impregnated collagen shields, liposomes, microspheres and iontophoresis.

Drugs may also be delivered intraocularly either by direct injection or by insertion of a slow release drug delivery implant device [1] but to date this has not been used in "high risk" cases of corneal graft rejection.

Drug-Based Immunosuppressant Therapy

Since systemic steroids were first shown to be useful for prevention and treatment of solid organ transplant rejection (for review see [2]), many attempts have been made to find more effective and safer drugs primarily because high dose prolonged steroid use was found to be associated with many side effects including fatal opportunistic infections. This has applied also to corneal graft rejection [3], but to a lesser extent since topical steroids have long been known to be effective in controlling rejection and were not associated with significant systemic side effects [4]. However, control of rejection in "high risk" grafts is not possible solely with topical steroids in many cases, and despite lower doses systemic steroids continued to have a significant toxicity. Accordingly, experimental studies have explored the therapeutic potential of several alternative systemic immunosuppressive drugs. These include azathioprine, cyclosporin, FK506, mycophenolate, and many others. Early experimental studies in rabbits showed that azathiporine was effective as a steroid sparing agent [3, 5] but this drug is known also to have significant side effects especially on bone marrow function [2].

Cyclosporin

Cyclosporin has been used for control of intraocular inflammation since the early 1980s when it was found to be effective in the control of experimental autoimmune uveoretinitis (for review see [6]). Since then it has been used both experimentally and clinically for control of corneal graft rejection but there is some controversy over its effectiveness. In the main, instances where it has been found not to be effective have been where there has been insufficient dosing or duration or there has been poor case selection. Cyclosporin is a calcineurin phospahatase inhibitor and blocks production of IL-2 via inhibition of the transcription factor, NFAT which functions via calcineurin induction [7]. Its mode of action is similar to other calcineurin inhibitors such as FK506.

Experimentally, cyclosporin is very effective in control of graft rejection in rabbits, rats and mice. Cyclosporin in most experiments appeared only to be active while administered i.e. it does not induce graft tolerance, nor was it effective prophylactically [8–12]. However, in one experiment of "high risk" grafts in rabbits CsA prevented graft rejection indefinitely (>180 days) after a 30-day course of treatment from the time of grafting [13]. In rats, CsA appeared to delay infiltration of MHC class II positive cells and macrophages into the iris as well as induce changes in the peripheral lymph node T cells but these corresponded with the overall delay in graft rejection [10, 14, 15].

Side effects are a significant problem clinically and many attempts have been made to apply the drug directly to the eye. In fact one of the original experiments demonstrated the drug's effectiveness when administered as a retrobulbar injection in a rabbit model [16]. Considerable inventiveness in ocular drug delivery systems has been applied including direct topical application of different formulations, impregnation of collagen shields, encapsulation in liposomes and microspheres, slow release extraocular drug delivery systems and others [17–30]. In general although there have been some favourable experimental studies the high hydrophobicity of the drug prevents its penetration into the cornea and the eye and an effective suitable local formulation for human clinical use is awaited.

FK506 (tacrolimus)

FK506, generally known as tacrolimus, is also a calcineurin inhibitor but has a different side effect profile to CsA [7]. Since it was first discovered in 1985, it has been used widely in solid organ transplantation including experimental corneal graft [31]. The drug was found to be as effective as CsA in a rat model but like CsA FK506 was only effective during the period of administration. On cessation of either drug, the graft rejection process was initiated [32]. In a xenograft model of corneal graft rejection, FK506 together with antiadhesion molecule therapy seemed to have a beneficial effect (see below).

Topical and subconjunctival FK506 therapy has also been evaluated in rat and rabbit models of keratoplasty and seems to have a beneficial effect while applied [33–35].

Few studies have been reported in human corneal grafts but it does appear to have value [36].

Mycophenolate mofetil

Mycophenolate mofetil (Cellcept, MMF) has been an important addition to the immunosuppression armamentarium for solid organ grafts since it was reintroduced in the early 1990s in a new metabolizable formulation [37]. Cellcept is a relatively selective inhibitor of T and B cell proliferation and adhesion through noncompetitive, reversible inhibition of inosine monophosphate dehydrogenase, an enzyme required for DNA synthesis at the guanine oligonucleotide level [38]. Its profile of side effects is significantly different from the calcineurin inhibitors and it is now being used in several other autoimmune and immune-mediated conditions [39].

In a rat model of corneal graft MMF had a beneficial effect when given preoperatively and postoperatively but higher doses were required to have an effect in the postoperative period [40]. In combination with CsA there appeared to be a significantly beneficial effect over either drug alone [41].

Other drugs

Several other immunosuppressive drugs have been tested experimentally but none have been shown to have a particular advantage over existing immunosuppressants sufficient to merit clinical development for corneal graft. These include drugs such as leflunamide [42, 43], deoxyspergaulin [44], misopristol [45] and rapamycin (Sirolimus) [46, 47].

Newer drugs

Several new drugs of interest are in developmental stages and some are in clinical trials in other types of solid organ transplantation. These include SDZ RAD (everolimus, Certican), a derivative of rapamycin, which is a novel macrolide immunosuppressant [48]. Its mechanism of action is to block alloantigen-induced T cell activation mediated by IL-2 receptor-driven p70-S6 kinase signalling which is downstream of calcineurin function. Thus it can act synergistically with CsA and FK506. It has been shown to be effective in this regime in rat kidney allograft survival [48] as well as corneal graft [46, 47].

Another new drug which may have value in corneal graft rejection is FTY720 which appears to function by inhibition of lymphocyte trafficking. This drug is currently under clinical trial in other forms of solid organ transplantation [49]. Like FTY720, triptolide is a drug which has been identified as a component of traditional Chinese medicine and has promising anti-inflammatory and anti-graft-rejection potential but has not yet been used in corneal graft studies [50]. Other interesting potential therapies include bovine seminal ribonuclease and urocanic acid [51, 52]. In addition, attention has been drawn to the anti-inflammatory and immunologic properties of statins, which are in widespread use as cholesterol-lowering agents [53].

Molecular Immunointervention

The extensive knowledge on molecular interactions in the immune response has led to a wide variety of approaches to modulate immunity. These include inhibition of CD4, CD8, TCR, costimulatory molecules, adhesion molecules, chemokines, and inflammatory mediators of the innate immune response amongst many others. Inhibition of specific molecules using polyclonal and monoclonal antibodies, receptor-targeted fusion proteins and genetically modified mice have been the main methods of investigation. In addition, the use of more "broad-spectrum" reagents such as rabbit anti-human thymocyte globulin (thymoglobulin) as adjuncts to inhibit T cell function generally has been found to be valuable in both solid organ and bone marrow transplantation in part because of the reduced likelihood of monospecific anti-idiotype reactions which may occur with other monoclonal antibody therapy [54]. The extensive literature on immunointervention in solid organ transplantation generally has been reviewed recently [55].

Several of these molecules have been explored in corneal graft rejection. Because of its relatively small size, pretreatment of the donor cornea with immunobiological reagents has been relatively straightforward and has been an adopted method for many years [56, 57].

Costimulation blockade

The number of costimulatory molecules known to be involved in T cell activation and regulation is increasing continually. CD40:CD154 interactions are important mediators of the second signal in immunity and inhibition of CD40 via anti-CD154 antibody significantly prolongs corneal allograft survival in mice but the effect does not induce sustained graft tolerance since rejection occurs when the administration of the antibody is terminated [58, 59]. Interestingly, even if the CD40 pathway is permanently impaired as in CD40 KO mice, graft rejection still occurs indicating that alternative costimulatory pathways are induced for priming to the allograft (Kuffová *et al.*, in preparation).

Blockade of the B7 costimulatory pathway using a CTLA-4 Ig fusion protein also prolongs corneal graft survival but only under certain circumstances. For instance incubation of high dose rabbit donor corneas with anti-CTLA4-Ig fails to prevent rejection, while lower doses of the fusion protein are effective [60]. This may be in part because CTLA-4 has a more significant role in T cell regulation, which occurs later during T cell activation. Thus high doses of the fusion protein may permit the protein to persist in an active state for longer in the anterior chamber and thus prevent the later downregulation of T cells which occurs naturally. Generally similar results were observed with topically applied CTLA4-Ig in a murine model of graft rejection [61] and have been confirmed more recently using both fusion protein pretreatment of the donor and transfection with CTLA4-expressing adenovirus [62].

T cell blockade

CD4+ T cells have been identified as the major cell type mediating corneal graft rejection as part of the paradigm implicating indirect rather than direct allorecognition in this process. Blocking antibodies to CD4+ T cells were found to prolong graft survival whereas blockade of CD8 mechanisms either by antibodies or by use of CD8 KO mice had essentially no effect on allograft survival [63–67]. CD4+ T cells are important in corneal xenograft rejection also [68] but CD8+ T cells may also play a role here [69] (see Chapter 7).

Inhibition of the TCR in the rat cornea graft model using the R73 antibody has proved to be effective in prolonging graft survival but by significantly different margins depending on the strain combination [70].

Antiadhesion molecule

Blockade of adhesion molecules has been investigated in several occasions in animal models both systemically and topically. The mode of action is not entirely clear since some adhesion molecules such as LFA-1 are also involved in the initial stages of T cell activation during antigen presentation as well as later in the egress of cells from the secondary lymphoid tissue as well as ingress into the tissue. Inhibition of LFA-1 but not ICAM-1 in isolation delays allograft rejection [71]. In a rat to mouse corneal xenograft model, antibodies to LFA-1, the leukocyte ligand for ICAM-1 and -3 on endothelial cells, has a minimal effect when used in isolation but is considerably more effective when used in combination with immunosuppressant drugs such as FK 506 [72] and despergauline [73]. Inhibition of VLA-4, particularly in combination with antibody to LFA-1 inhibits both immune responsiveness and corneal allograft rejection [74, 75]. A humanized anti-LFA-1 is available for clinical use but has not yet been assessed for prevention of corneal graft rejection [76].

Anticytokine/chemokine

Blockade of cytokines such as IL-1α by its receptor antagonist [77–79] and TNF-α topically as well as systemically, has also been shown to be effective in delaying graft rejection and most recently IL-15 has been added to this list of possible therapeutic targets (Kuffová *et al.*, in preparation). Part of this effect appears to be mediated by preventing chemokine expression [80]. Inhibition of graft rejection by IL-1ra appears to be mediated purely by its effects on the inflammatory response and not by any effect on induction of an ACAID-like tolerance response [77].

Anti-innate immunity

Much of the damaging effect of the innate immune response is mediated by macrophages and early studies in a rat corneal graft model showed that depletion of macrophages locally by subconjunctival injection of liposomes, containing the macrophage specific drug clodronate, led to an indefinite prolongation of corneal graft survival [81]. Studies of CTL activity indicated that despite local application, immunosuppressive effects were detected systemically [82] and particularly in the draining submandibular lymph nodes [83]. Much of the effect appeared to be mediated by reduction of inflammatory cytokines as might be expected [84].

Gene Therapy

The cornea offers an excellent opportunity to investigate the possibility of gene therapy approaches to the prevention of graft rejection.

Transfection of the donor graft endothelial cells, which are the main target of attack by the host, with vectors expressing one or more immunoregulatory molecules would seem at first sight to be an ideal means to inhibit the immune response. One of the first molecules to be tested in this fashion was CTLA-4 [62]. However, local adenoviral-meditated expression of CTLA-4 had little effect on graft survival compared to systemic expression. This is most likely explained by the site of action of this regulatory molecule which would be more active during priming in the draining lymph node than in the effector stage at the site of immune attack (see Chapter 6).

A more dramatic effect was observed with IL-10-transfected endothelial cells in an outbred model of sheep corneal graft [85] (Figure 10.1). Effectiveness of this treatment depends critically on the duration of expression of the transfectant which was shown to be about 28 days by in vitro testing. The aim would be indefinite constitutive expression. Treatment of

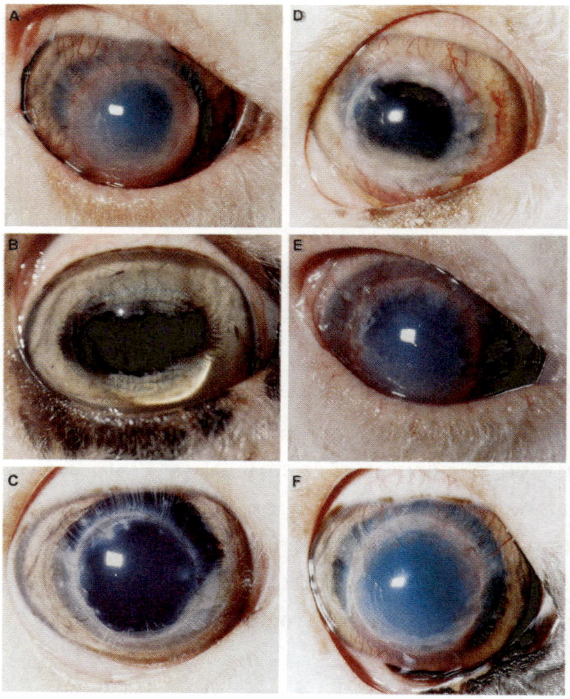

Figure 10.1 Full-thickness penetrating keratoplasty in the sheep. (**A, E, F**) Control untreated eyes showing rejection (corneal opacification) of donor grafts; (**B, C, D**) accepted, clear corneal grafts in which donor grafts were pretreated by transfection with IL-10 plasmid vector prior to grafting.

ocular surface disease and graft rejection itself has been suggested by transfection of IL-1ra [86] or IL-10 [87].

Conclusion

There are many novel potential modalities for investigating and developing new therapies for prevention of corneal graft rejection. Probably the most important factor is application to clinically relevant models. While immunomodulation of corneal graft rejection in the naïve animal is important in understanding the immune mechanisms, most human corneal grafts which undergo rejection are "high risk" and application of new therapies to models of "high risk" rejection would seem to be a useful approach.

References

1. Bourlais CL *et al.* Ophthalmic drug delivery systems—recent advances. *Prog Retin Eye Res* 1998; 17(1): 33.
2. Ponticelli C, Tarantino A and Vegeto A. Renal transplantation: past, present and future. *J Nephrol* 1999; 12 Suppl 2: S105.
3. D'Amico RA and Castroviejo R. Suppression of the immune response in keratoplasty. *Am J Ophthalmol* 1969; 68(5): 829.
4. Barraquer J. Keratoplasty and keratoprosthesis. Pocklington Memorial Lecture delivered at the Royal College of Surgeons of England on 5th May, 1966. *Ann R Coll Surg Engl* 1967; 40(2): 71.
5. Leibowitz HM and Elliott JH. Chemotherapeutic immunosuppression of the corneal graft reaction: II. Combined systemic antimetabolite and topical corticosteroid therapy. *Arch Ophthalmol* 1966; 76(3): 338.
6. Nussenblatt RB. Bench to bedside: new approaches to the immunotherapy of uveitic disease. *Int Rev Immunol* 2002; 21(2–3): 273.
7. Jorgensen KA, Koefoed-Nielsen PB and Karamperis N. Calcineurin phosphatase activity and immunosuppression: a review on the role of calcineurin phosphatase activity and the immunosuppressive effect of cyclosporin A and tacrolimus. *Scand J Immunol* 2003; 57(2): 93.
8. Bouchard CS, Kappil JC and Duffner L. The role of systemic cyclosporine dosing schedule on corneal allograft survival in the rat model. *Curr Eye Res* 1995; 14(5): 421.
9. Claerhout I *et al.* The effect of duration and timing of systemic cyclosporine therapy on corneal allograft survival in a rat model. *Graefes Arch Clin Exp Ophthalmol* 2001; 239(2): 152.
10. Coupland SE, Krause L and Hoffmann F. The influence of penetrating keratoplasty and cyclosporin A therapy on MHC class II (Ia)-positive cells in the rat iris and choroid. *Graefes Arch Clin Exp Ophthalmol* 1996; 234(2): 116.

11. Herbort CP *et al.* Penetrating keratoplasty in the rat: a model for the study of immunosuppressive treatment of graft rejection. *Jpn J Ophthalmol* 1989; 33(2): 212.
12. Zhang EP *et al.* The effect of corticosteroid and cyclosporin A on murine corneal allograft rejection. *Graefes Arch Clin Exp Ophthalmol* 2000; 238(6): 525.
13. Rehany U and Waisman M. Suppression of corneal allograft rejection by systemic cyclosporine-A in heavily vascularized rabbit corneas following alkali burns. *Cornea* 1994; 13(5): 447.
14. Krause L, Coupland SE and Hoffmann F. The behaviour of ED1- and ED2-positive cells in the rat iris and choroid following penetrating keratoplasty and cyclosporin A therapy. *Graefes Arch Clin Exp Ophthalmol* 1996; 234 Suppl 1: S149.
15. Klebe S *et al.* Flow-cytometric analysis of peripheral lymphocytes in the rat following penetrating keratoplasty and immunosuppressive treatment. *Ger J Ophthalmol* 1996; 5(3): 137.
16. Salisbury JD and Gebhardt BM. Suppression of corneal allograft rejection by cyclosporin A. *Arch Ophthalmol* 1981; 99(9): 1640.
17. Apel A *et al.* A subconjunctival degradable implant for cyclosporine delivery in corneal transplant therapy. *Curr Eye Res* 1995; 14(8): 659.
18. Belin MW, Bouchard CS and Phillips TM. Update on topical cyclosporin A: background, immunology, and pharmacology. *Cornea* 1990; 9(3): 184.
19. de Rojas Silva MV *et al.* Efficacy of subconjunctival cyclosporin-containing microspheres on keratoplasty rejection in the rabbit. *Graefes Arch Clin Exp Ophthalmol* 1999; 237(10): 840.
20. Juberias JR *et al.* Efficacy of topical cyclosporine-loaded nanocapsules on keratoplasty rejection in the rat. *Curr Eye Res* 1998; 17(1): 39.
21. Kana JS *et al.* Rabbit corneal allograft survival following topical administration of cyclosporin A. *Invest Ophthalmol Vis Sci* 1982; 22(5): 686.
22. Mahlberg K *et al.* Prevention of experimental corneal allograft rejection in rabbits using cyclosporin-collagen shields. *Graefes Arch Clin Exp Ophthalmol* 1991; 229(1): 69.
23. Mahlberg K, Uusitalo RJ and Oksala O. Prevention of high risk corneal graft rejection using cyclosporine A (CsA) incorporated into a collagen matrix. *Ocul Immunol Inflamm* 1997; 5(2): 101.
24. Milani JK *et al.* Prolongation of corneal allograft survival with liposome-encapsulated cyclosporine in the rat eye. *Ophthalmology* 1993; 100(6): 890.
25. Shi W, Xie L and Wang S. Prolongation of corneal allograft survival in mice with a cyclosporine drug delivery system implant. *Chung Hua Yen Ko Tsa Chih* 2002; 38(8): 502.
26. Williams DL. A comparative approach to topical cyclosporine therapy. *Eye* 1997; 11 (Pt 4): 453.
27. Williams KA, Erickson SA, and Coster DJ. Topical steroid, cyclosporin A, and the outcome of rat corneal allografts. *Br J Ophthalmol* 1987; 71(3): 239.
28. Williams KA *et al.* A comparison of the effects of topical cyclosporine and topical steroid on rabbit corneal allograft rejection. *Transplantation* 1985; 39(3): 242.
29. Xie L *et al.* Prolongation of corneal allograft survival using cyclosporine in a polylactide-co-glycolide polymer. *Cornea* 2001; 20(7): 748.
30. Zhao JC and Jin XY. Local therapy of corneal allograft rejection with cyclosporine. *Am J Ophthalmol* 1995; 119(2): 189.
31. Nishi M *et al.* Effects of the immunosuppressant FK506 on a penetrating keratoplasty rejection model in the rat. *Invest Ophthalmol Vis Sci* 1993; 34(8): 2477.

32. Reis A *et al.* A comparative investigation of FK506 and cyclosporin A in murine corneal transplantation. *Graefes Arch Clin Exp Ophthalmol* 1998; 236(10): 785.
33. Minamoto A *et al.* Suppression of corneal graft rejection by subconjunctival injection of FK-506 in a rat model of penetrating keratoplasty. *Jpn J Ophthalmol* 1995; 39(1): 12.
34. Mills RA *et al.* Topical FK-506 prevents experimental corneal allograft rejection. *Cornea* 1995; 14(2): 157.
35. Okada K *et al.* Effect of FK 506 administered topically versus intramuscularly on suppression of the corneal immune reaction in rats. *Ophthalmologica* 1996; 210(3): 175.
36. Sloper CM, Powell RJ and Dua HS. Tacrolimus (FK506) in the management of high-risk corneal and limbal grafts. *Ophthalmology* 2001; 108(10): 1838.
37. Collier SJ. Immunosuppressive drugs. *Curr Opin Immunol* 1989; 2(6): 854.
38. McMurray RW and Harisdangkul V. Mycophenolate mofetil: selective T cell inhibition. *Am J Med Sci* 2002; 323(4): 194.
39. Moder KG. Mycophenolate mofetil: new applications for this immunosuppressant. *Ann Allergy Asthma Immunol* 2003; 90(1):15; quiz 20, 78.
40. Reis A *et al.* Beneficial effect of preoperative mycophenolate mofetil in murine corneal transplantation. *Transpl Int* 1999; 12(5): 341.
41. Reis A *et al.* Effect of mycophenolate mofetil, cyclosporin A, and both in combination in a murine corneal graft rejection model. *Br J Ophthalmol* 1998; 82(6): 700.
42. Coupland SE *et al.* Leflunomide therapy following penetrating keratoplasty in the rat. *Graefes Arch Clin Exp Ophthalmol* 1994; 232(10): 622.
43. Niederkorn JY *et al.* Promotion of corneal allograft survival with leflunomide. *Invest Ophthalmol Vis Sci* 1994; 35(10): 3783.
44. Holland EJ *et al.* Suppression of graft rejection using 15-deoxyspergualin in the allogeneic rat penetrating keratoplasty model. *Cornea* 1994; 13(1): 28.
45. Olsen TW, Gothard TW and Holland EJ. Misoprostol with cyclosporin A prolongs corneal allograft survival in an animal model. *Cornea* 1996; 15(1): 76.
46. Reis A *et al.* RAD, a new immunosuppressive macrolide in murine corneal transplantation. *Graefes Arch Clin Exp Ophthalmol* 2001; 239(9): 689.
47. Reis A *et al.* Synergism of RAD and cyclosporin A in prevention of acute rat corneal allograft rejection. *Cornea* 2002; 21(1): 81.
48. Nashan B. Early clinical experience with a novel rapamycin derivative. *Ther Drug Monit* 2002; 24(1): 53.
49. Brinkmann V and Lynch KR. FTY720: targeting G-protein-coupled receptors for sphingosine 1-phosphate in transplantation and autoimmunity. *Curr Opin Immunol* 2002; 14(5): 569.
50. Chen BJ. Triptolide, a novel immunosuppressive and anti-inflammatory agent purified from a Chinese herb Tripterygium wilfordii Hook F. *Leuk Lymphoma* 2001; 42(3): 253.
51. Filipec M *et al.* Immunosuppressive effect of bovine seminal ribonuclease on a model of corneal transplantation in rabbit. *Graefes Arch Clin Exp Ophthalmol* 1996; 234(9): 586.
52. Filipec M *et al.* The effect of urocanic acid on graft rejection in an experimental model of orthotopic corneal transplantation in rabbits. *Graefes Arch Clin Exp Ophthalmol* 1998; 236(1): 65.
53. Mach F. Statins as immunomodulators. *Transpl Immunol* 2002; 9(2–4): 197.

54. Regan J *et al.* Characterization of anti-thymoglobulin, anti-Atgam and anti-OKT3 IgG antibodies in human serum with an 11-min ELISA. *Transpl Immunol* 1997; 5(1): 49.
55. Hong JC and Kahan BD. Immunosuppressive agents in organ transplantation: past, present, and future. *Semin Nephrol* 2000; 20(2): 108.
56. Chandler JW. Immunologic protection of rabbit corneal allografts: prolonged survival of allografts pretreated with homologous antibody against transplantation antigens. *Invest Ophthalmol* 1976; 15(3): 213.
57. Smolin G. Suppression of corneal graft reaction by antilymphocyte serum. *Arch Ophthalmol* 1968; 79(5): 603.
58. Zhang EP, Bulfone-Paus S and Hoffmann F. Immunomodulation after keratoplasty by CTL4-Ig and anti-CD154 antibodies. *Ophthalmologe* 2002; 99(3): 183.
59. Qian Y *et al.* Blockade of CD40-CD154 costimulatory pathway promotes survival of allogeneic corneal transplants. *Invest Ophthalmol Vis Sci* 2001; 42(5): 987.
60. Gebhardt BM *et al.* Protection of corneal allografts by CTLA4-Ig. *Cornea* 1999; 18(3): 314.
61. Hoffmann F *et al.* Inhibition of corneal allograft reaction by CTLA4-Ig. *Graefes Arch Clin Exp Ophthalmol* 1997; 235(8): 535.
62. Comer RM *et al.* Effect of administration of CTLA4-Ig as protein or cDNA on corneal allograft survival. *Invest Ophthalmol Vis Sci* 2002; 43(4): 1095.
63. He YG, Ross J and Niederkorn JY. Promotion of murine orthotopic corneal allograft survival by systemic administration of anti-CD4 monoclonal antibody. *Invest Ophthalmol Vis Sci* 1991; 32(10): 2723.
64. Ayliffe W *et al.* Prolongation of rat corneal graft survival by treatment with anti-CD4 monoclonal antibody. *Br J Ophthalmol* 1992; 76(10): 602.
65. Hašková Z *et al.* CD4+ T cells are critical for corneal, but not skin, allograft rejection. *Transplantation* 2000; 69(4): 483.
66. Hegde S and Niederkorn JY. The role of cytotoxic T lymphocytes in corneal allograft rejection. *Invest Ophthalmol Vis Sci* 2000; 41(11): 3341.
67. Yamada J, Ksander BR, and Streilein JW. Cytotoxic T cells play no essential role in acute rejection of orthotopic corneal allografts in mice. *Invest Ophthalmol Vis Sci* 2001; 42(2): 386.
68. Tanaka K, Sonoda K and Streilein JW. Acute rejection of orthotopic corneal xenografts in mice depends on CD4(+) T cells and self-antigen-presenting cells. *Invest Ophthalmol Vis Sci* 2001; 42(12): 2878.
69. Higuchi R and Streilein JW. CD8+ T cell-mediated delayed rejection of orthotopic guinea pig cornea grafts in mice deficient in CD4+ T cells. *Invest Ophthalmol Vis Sci* 2003; 44(1): 175.
70. Yamagami S *et al.* Suppression of allograft rejection with anti-alphabeta T cell receptor antibody in rat corneal transplantation. *Transplantation* 1999; 67(4): 600.
71. He Y *et al.* Effect of LFA-1 and ICAM-1 antibody treatment on murine corneal allograft survival. *Invest Ophthalmol Vis Sci* 1994; 35(8): 3218.
72. Yamagami S *et al.* Mechanism of concordant corneal xenograft rejection in mice: synergistic effects of anti-leukocyte function-associated antigen-1 monoclonal antibody and FK506. *Transplantation* 1997; 64(1): 42.
73. Yamagami S *et al.* Prolongation of corneal xenograft survival with deoxyspergualin and anti-LFA-1 monoclonal antibody. *Transplant Proc* 1997; 29(4): 2288.

74. Hori J *et al.* Specific immunosuppression of corneal allograft rejection by combination of anti-VLA-4 and anti-LFA-1 monoclonal antibodies in mice. *Exp Eye Res* 1997; 65(1): 89.
75. Hori J *et al.*. Effect of monoclonal antibody to VLA-4 on corneal allograft survival in mice. *Transplant Proc* 1996; 28(3): 1990.
76. Dedrick RL, Walicke P and Garovoy M. Anti-adhesion antibodies efalizumab, a humanized anti-CD11a monoclonal antibody. *Transpl Immunol* 2002; 9(2–4): 181.
77. Yamada J *et al.* Interleukin-1 receptor antagonist therapy and induction of anterior chamber-associated immune deviation-type tolerance after corneal transplantation. *Invest Ophthalmol Vis Sci* 2000; 41(13): 4203.
78. Yamada J *et al.* Interleukin 1 receptor antagonist suppresses allosensitization in corneal transplantation. *Arch Ophthalmol* 1998; 116(10): 1351.
79. Dana MR, Yamada J and Streilein JW. Topical interleukin 1 receptor antagonist promotes corneal transplant survival. *Transplantation* 1997; 63(10): 1501.
80. Qian Y *et al.* Topical soluble tumor necrosis factor receptor type I suppresses ocular chemokine gene expression and rejection of allogeneic corneal transplants. *Arch Ophthalmol* 2000; 118(12): 1666.
81. Van der Veen G *et al.* Prevention of corneal allograft rejection in rats treated with subconjunctival injections of liposomes containing dichloromethylene diphosphonate. *Invest Ophthalmol Vis Sci* 1994; 35(9): 3505.
82. Van der Veen G *et al.* Cytotoxic T lymphocytes and antibodies after orthotropic penetrating keratoplasty in rats treated with dichloromethylene diphosphonate encapsulated liposomes. *Curr Eye Res* 1998; 17(10): 1018.
83. Slegers TP *et al.* Effect of macrophage depletion on immune effector mechanisms during corneal allograft rejection in rats. *Invest Ophthalmol Vis Sci* 2000; 41(8): 2239.
84. Torres PF *et al.* Changes in cytokine mRNA levels in experimental corneal allografts after local clodronate-liposome treatment. *Invest Ophthalmol Vis Sci* 1999; 40(13): 3194.
85. Klebe S *et al.* Prolongation of sheep corneal allograft survival by *ex vivo* transfer of the gene encoding interleukin-10. *Transplantation* 2001; 71(9): 1214.
86. Moore J E *et al.* The inflammatory milieu associated with conjunctivalized cornea and its alteration with IL-1 RA gene therapy. *Invest Ophthalmol Vis Sci* 2002; 43(9): 2905.
87. Shen J *et al.* *Ex vivo* adenovirus mediated gene transfection of human conjunctival epithelium. *Br J Ophthalmol* 2001; 85(7): 861.

11

Immunosuppression for Human Corneal Graft Rejection

Introduction

There are many reasons for the high rate of success of "low risk" human corneal grafts, some of which are the avascularity and small size of the graft, and possible immune privilege (see Chapter 6). In "high risk" patients the picture is different. In patients who have a compromised corneal surface or suffer additional systemic immunological disease, the outcome after corneal transplantation is poor [1, 2]. Despite improved donor tissue management, better understanding and earlier recognition of the varied clinical manifestations of corneal graft rejection, and modern medical treatment, corneal graft rejection remains the major cause of allograft failure. The reported incidence of graft rejection in "low risk" patients is 15–35% [3–5]. In this group early recognition of the rejection process, and rapid and aggressive treatment can save the majority of the grafts. On the other hand for grafts at "high risk" of rejection the outcome of corneal graft is poor even if rejection is treated as aggressively as possible [1]. In the first three years post graft, the proportion of eyes with failure from rejection is 30% for the ABO-incompatible group and 16% for the ABO-compatible group [1], which is a poorer outcome than that observed for some other solid organ grafts [6]. Most corneal graft rejection occurs within 6 months of transplantation and the speed and severity of the rejection episode correlates with the degree of previous vascularization of the cornea [7].

Immediate Postoperative Therapy for Corneal Grafts

Part of the reason for the success of nonmatched corneal grafts may be due to the standard practice of instituting topical steroid therapy routinely after graft and continuing this therapy for a variable period of several weeks, then gradually tapering off treatment. In addition, risk factors for initiating rejection such as loose sutures and foci of corneal neovascularization can be appropriately managed in a prophylactic way.

Topical corticosteroid drops such as 1% prednisolone acetate or 0.1% dexamethazone sodium are used routinely for every case in the early post-operative period. They are usually used 4–6 times per day and tapered over several (6 months) months unless the patient is at "high risk" of corneal rejection. In such cases they are used more frequently and for a longer period [8–10]. If the patient develops increased inflammation in the anterior chamber of the eye, keratic precipitates on the cornea or increased thickness of the graft, the topical steroid treatment is usually increased.

Patients with "high risk" grafts may be treated prophylactically with non-steroidal immunosuppressants. The drug regime for these therapies is similar to the use of these drugs to control rejection (see below).

Management of Graft Rejection

The management of the rejection episode depends on the patient, the severity of the inflammation, the timing of recognition of the rejection episode and whether the graft is "low risk" or "high risk".

Indications for treatment

The indications for treatment are the signs and symptoms of rejection. The earlier these are recognized and treated the more successful is the treatment. Rejection in "low risk" grafts occurs usually some time after cessation of topical steroid therapy and is triggered often by some nonspecific insult, including unexpected events such as vaccination for influenza [11].

Rejection in "high risk" grafts may occur despite topical therapy and may require systemic immunosuppression (see below) to prevent it.

Any of the three corneal layers can initiate a rejection response. Clinically, in the human each of the layers exhibits recognizable features during rejection (see Chapter 3). These clinical features are also seen in animal corneal grafting models (see Chapter 8). The symptoms and signs of ongoing corneal rejection are usually mild and nonspecific at the beginning of a rejection episode. The mild pain, decrease of vision, "red" eye and photophobia are the most common symptoms and all patients post corneal transplantation should be made aware of these important symptoms by appropriate counselling. Kamp *et al.* found that in a group of "high risk" patients, nearly 70% of graft rejection episodes were preceded by patient symptoms and only 30% of allograft rejections were identified on routine clinical examination [12]. However, the sensitivity and specificity of patient symptoms as an indicator of graft rejection was poor. Despite this, patient symptoms cannot be ignored, and the symptomatic patient must be evaluated to rule out a rejection episode [12].

Topical steroid therapy

Some episodes of allograft rejection can be reversed by topical steroids if prompt and aggressive treatment is initiated. This usually takes the form of intensive drop application of a high strength steroid preparation such as hourly 0.1% dexamethazone sodium or 1.0% prednisolone acetate. Typically, the majority of graft rejection episodes are reversed by this treatment in a few days and do not lead to graft failure [13]. However, even with current aggressive medical management aimed at prevention and early recognition of graft rejection especially in the "high risk" patients, the rejection process once initiated usually leads to corneal graft failure and ultimately loss of vision. For this reason, some surgeons treat all rejection episodes with a short course of systemic steroids. The best treatment of rejection is prevention, and early recognition of "high risk" clinical features preoperatively. In addition, patient education on the importance of recognizing the symptoms of graft rejection and the possibility of initiating early and aggressive therapy immediately after recognition of the rejection process, help to minimise these effects [14].

Systemic steroids

Corticosteroids remain the treatment of choice for more severe acute rejection episodes. The routes of administration include periocular, oral, and intravenous. Periocular steroids have recently been shown to act in part by systemic absorption and are therefore included as such here [15]. There is continuing controversy concerning topical vs oral steroid therapy even for severe acute rejection episodes. For instance, topical 1% prednisolone acetate was preferred over subconjunctival or systemic corticosteroids by the Castroviejo Society [16]. In addition, there is no consensus over the most effective route for systemic steroids. Hill *et al.* demonstrated in a prospective study that 500 mg intravenous methylprednisolone in a single dose was more effective and better tolerated than daily oral prednisolone (60–80 mg) when combined with topical steroids in corneal graft rejection [17]. When patients were treated with systemic steroids within 8 days of the onset of symptoms, the survival rate of grafts was 92% vs 55%. Hill *et al.* also found that a second dose of methylprednisolone at 24 or 48 hours had no advantage over a single dose [18]. In the study by Hudde *et al.* for treatment of graft rejection, additional systemic treatment with 500 mg methylprednisolone yielded no significant benefit over intensive topical corticosteroid alone [19]. Graft survival following treatment of a rejection episode with local corticosteroid treatment alone is good in those patients without other risk factors for graft failure.

Long term immunosuppression for control of corneal graft rejection

Recipients of grafts at "high risk" of corneal rejection require more long term immunosuppressive therapy but there are several difficulties in deciding the best strategy. Firstly, prolonged use of systemic steroids is not recommended because of the inevitable development of side effects, including the high incidence of intolerable weight gain and the psychological side effects. However, limited studies of second line drugs have been reported. In addition, no universally accepted definition of the "high risk" recipient exists: a previous history of graft failure, corneal opacity due to herpetic infection and any heavily vascularized recipient bed are all regarded as "high risk". The variability in criteria means different treatment regimens are difficult to compare and evaluate. Studies of degree of vascularization using univariate and multivariate survival analysis suggest that recipient corneas can be divided into low, medium and high risk, depending on the number of quadrants of vascularization (avascular, 1–2 quadrants and 3+ quadrants respectively). This wider classification would make the design and comparison of treatment regimens more consistent and reliable.

In "high risk" cases, therefore, two different therapeutic courses arise: (1) In preparation for grafting, the patient may receive a "cover" of steroids for the perioperative period while also being placed on prophylactic immunosuppression with, for instance, a calcineurin inhibitor such as cyclosporin (CsA) [20]. (2) When managing rejection episodes in a "high risk" graft in which the patient is not already on immunosuppression, a severe reaction involving the endothelium requires initial control of the rejection episode with rapid acting steroids. In this circumstance, instead of oral steroids, it is preferable to use an intravenous "pulse" of 500 mg methylprednisolone: this is at least as effective as longer duration oral steroids, avoids prolonged medication, and may confer some long term benefit [1, 20]. At the same time the patient should be placed on a long term agent such as CsA or FK506.

Hill *et al.* found that in "high risk" keratoplasty, graft survival was greatly improved if systemic CsA was used in addition to systemic and topical steroids as compared to use of topical steroids alone [21]. It was also shown that the maximum effect was obtained if the cyclosporine was used for 12 months instead of 6 months, demonstrating a 93% vs 69% graft survival rate, respectively [22]. This improvement resulted from both a reduction in the incidence, and an increase in the reversal rate, of rejection episodes. The improvement continued after stopping CsA therapy, suggesting that some degree of immunological privilege had been re-established [22].

Others have found similar results with CsA. Oral CsA was used in addition to high dose intravenous pulse methylprednisolone in therapy of acute corneal graft rejection [23, 24]. This approach to the treatment of acute corneal graft rejection has been shown to be safe and effective in reversing the rejection process and also may protect the graft from subsequent episodes of allograft rejection [24]. The treatment with oral CsA in the prevention and treatment of immune graft rejection in heavily vascularized, repeated keratoplasties with "high risk" for failure was tested in a study by Rumelt *et al.* [25]. Systemic CsA in this study had a limited beneficial effect in preventing immune graft rejection in repeated corneal transplants in a highly vascularized corneal bed and required continuous use at significantly high doses to be effective. When immune graft rejection occurred in such regrafts, the prognosis was poor despite continuing aggressive medical treatment [25].

Systemic treatment with CsA was also used in patients who required central corneolimbal grafts [26]. Treatment with CsA was successful and sufficient for 14 eyes with severe stem cell deficiencies when used up to 20.6 months on average postoperatively. This new treatment principle promises long term rehabilitation for a majority of eyes with severe limbal stem cell deficiencies [26]. Unfortunately the systemic use of any immunosuppressive drugs brings significant side effects from which the development of tumours is the most serious [27]. Skin and lip cancers, lymphomas and Kaposi's sarcomas are the main types of cancer in immunosuppressed patients. A number of risk factors have been identified, such as reactivation of latent viral infections, prolonged treatment regimen and a high level of immunosuppression [28]. Therefore, careful preoperative evaluation of patients for systemic immunosuppressive treatment is important.

Problems with side effects have stimulated ophthalmologists to consider topical nonsteroidal immunosuppressive treatment. In the case of CsA, a topical preparation is available and has been reported to be effective in some cases [29, 30], reaching comparable or even higher concentrations in the anterior chamber and conjunctiva than after systemic treatment [31]. However, topical CsA also may have serious side effects for the eye, such as persistence of herpetic infectious keratitis [32]. In general, reactivation of herpetic keratitis and persistent superficial corneal defects are the major complications with use of topical CsA. Therefore, combination systemic antiviral treatment with topical CsA in cases of active, but also prophylactically in inactive herpetic keratitis would be beneficial for patients at risk.

Despite the extensive use of immunosuppressants in many types of solid organ transplantation, few other systemic immunosuppressive drugs have been tried for prevention or treatment of corneal graft rejection even in "high risk" cases. The systemic use of tacrolimus (FK 506), another calcineurin inhibitor, was tested for its efficacy in controlling and preventing immune rejection episodes in patients with "high risk" corneal and limbal grafts [33–35]. In these studies almost 50% of recipients with the "high risk" of rejection remained clear with no signs of side effects of tacrolimus.

Mycophenolate mofetil (MMF), a purine synthesis inhibitor (see Chapter 10), has also recently been tested and compared to CsA in a series of studies from one centre [36–38]. Systemic treatment with MMF proved to be at least as safe as CsA and was recommended as an alternative to CsA for systemic immunosuppression after full-thickness penetrating keratoplasty.

Azathioprine and cyclophosphamide have been frequently used as immunosuppressive drugs in the past [39]. Due to the potentially dangerous side effect of aplastic anaemia [40], today their use is restricted to refractory and recurrent cases of immune rejection as an adjunctive therapy in combination with other immunosuppresive drugs.

New therapeutic approaches

Promising and novel immunosuppressive drugs designed to prevent transplant rejection in other systems have been developed recently. Two monoclonal antibodies directed against the interleukin-2 (IL-2) receptor, daclizumab and basiliximab, have been shown to significantly reduce the incidence of acute rejection in pancreas–kidney allografts, without increasing adverse events [41, 42]. However, these have not been evaluated in corneal graft rejection as yet.

Due to its use in severe sight-threatening intraocular inflammation [43], the antileucocyte (anti-CD52w) monoclonal antibody CAMPATH-1H has been tried in a single reported case of corneal graft rejection with good effect [44]. Campath-1H is a depleting antibody and induces significant bone marrow suppression. However, it has proved to be extremely effective as an immunosuppressant in the treatment of a range of refractory ocular disorders, including corneal melts and rejection episodes [43, 44].

Sirolimus (rapamycin), an agent that inhibits T- and B-responses at a later stage in intracelluar signalling than CsA, has been shown to be synergistic with CsA in experimental and clinical studies [45, 46]. Ongoing clinical trials have reported that in renal transplantation high doses of sirolimus are as effective as CsA. SDZ-RAD, a derivative of sirolimus, is also under investigation (see Chapter 10).

Other very recently developed immunosuppressants, including FTY-720 and the recombinant cytokine IL-2PE40, are also showing promise in experimental studies (see Chapter 10). IL-12 PE40 was shown to prolong the survival of experimental corneal allografts and synergised with cyclosporin and sirolimus [47]. Gusperimus (deoxyspergualin), which inhibits IL-1 synthesis, was useful in reversing early and late acute rejection in clinical trials. A further potential approach is the use of antisense oligonucleotides directed against adhesion molecules such as intercellular adhesion molecule-1, an important molecule in rejection, and it gave encouraging results in preventing rejection of primate renal allografts [48]. Many other experimental approaches are currently being tested (see Chapter 10).

Conclusion

Corneal graft rejection at least in the first year is well managed in many cases with topical steroids, and rejection episodes if identified early enough can also be readily reversed in many situations. The main difficulty is the management of the "high risk" case and in particular the prophylactic care of the repeat graft. Reliable information from well-conducted prospective clinical trials is not available in corneal transplantation as it is for other organs.

In addition, while recognizing that there is considerable debate over many unresolved issues, attention to factors such as surgical technique (induction of innate immunity) and tissue and blood group matching (induction of adaptive immunity) are as important as the use of immunosuppressive drugs in achieving a good outcome.

There is no doubt, however, that the availability of new drugs, and the inventive therapeutic approaches they involve, will allow further reduction in the risk of rejection in organ transplantation generally. However, caution is warranted with their use in order to avoid the risks of over immunosuppression. Today excellent results in transplantation generally, can be obtained with the currently available drugs. Newer immunosuppressive schedules should be designed, not only to reduce the risk of rejection, but also to obtain a better therapeutic index that allows a further improvement of the graft survival while minimising the comorbidity and drug-related toxicity.

References

1. The collaborative corneal transplantation studies (CCTS): effectiveness of histocompatibility matching in high-risk corneal transplantation. The Collaborative Corneal Transplantation Studies Research Group. *Arch Ophthalmol* 1992; 110(10): 1392.
2. The Australian Corneal Graft Registry: 1990 to 1992 report. *Aust N Z J Ophthalmol* 1993; 21(2 Suppl): 1.
3. Claesson M, Armitage WJ, Fagerholm P and Stenevi U. Visual outcome in corneal grafts: a preliminary analysis of the Swedish Corneal Transplant Register. *Br J Ophthalmol* 2002; 86(2): 174.
4. Vail A, Gore SM, Bradley BA, Easty DL and Rogers CA. Corneal graft survival and visual outcome: a multicenter study. Corneal Transplant Follow-up Study Collaborators. *Ophthalmology* 1994; 101(1): 120.
5. Price FW Jr, Whitson WE and Marks RG. Graft survival in four common groups of patients undergoing penetrating keratoplasty. *Ophthalmology* 1991; 98(3): 322.
6. Williams KA, Muehlberg SM, Lewis RF and Coster DJ. How successful is corneal transplantation? A report from the Australian Corneal Graft Register. *Eye* 1995; 9(Pt 2): 219.
7. Khodadoust AA. The allograft reaction: the leading cause of late failure of clinical corneal grafts. In: Jones BR (ed.), *Corneal Graft Failure* (Ciba Foundation Symposium; Elsevier, Amsterdam, 1973), 151.
8. Barron BA. Penetrating Keratoplasty. In: Kaufman HE, Barron BA and McDonald MB, *The Cornea* (Butterworth-Heinemann, Boston, 1998), p. 838.

9. Barker NH, Henderson TR, Ross CA, Coster DJ and Williams KA. Current Australian practice in the prevention and management of corneal allograft rejection. *Clin Exp Ophthalmol* 2000; 28(5): 357.
10. Burdon MA and McDonnell P. A survey of corneal graft practice in the United Kingdom. *Eye* 1995; 9(Pt 6, Su): 6.
11. Solomon A and Frucht-Pery J. Bilateral simultaneous corneal graft rejection after influenza vaccination. *Am J Ophthalmol* 1996; 121(6): 708.
12. Kamp MT, Fink NE, Enger C, Maguire MG, Stark WJ and Stulting RD. Patient-reported symptoms associated with graft reactions in high-risk patients in the collaborative corneal transplantation studies. *Cornea* 1995; 14: 43.
13. Sit M, Weisbrod DJ, Naor J and Slomovic AR. Corneal graft outcome study. *Cornea* 2001; 20: 129.
14. Maguire MG, Stark WJ, Gottsch JD, Stulting RD, Sugar A, Fink NE and Schwartz A. Risk factors for corneal graft failure and rejection in the collaborative corneal transplantation studies. Collaborative Corneal Transplantation Studies Research Group. *Ophthalmology* 1994; 101: 1536.
15. Weitjens O, von der Sluijs FA, Schoemaker RC, Lentjes EGWM, Cohen A, Romijn, FPHTM and van Meurs JC. Peribulbar corticosteroid injection: vitreal and serum concentrations after dexamethasone disodium phosphate injection. *Am J Ophthalmol* 1997; 123: 358.
16. Rinne JR and Stulting RD. Current practices in the prevention and treatment of corneal graft rejection. *Cornea* 1992; 11: 326.
17. Hill JC, Maske R and Watson P. Corticosteroids in corneal graft rejection: oral versus single pulse therapy. *Ophthalmology* 1991; 98: 329.
18. Hill JC and Ivey A. Corticosteroids in corneal graft rejection: double versus single pulse therapy. *Cornea* 1994; 13(5): 383.
19. Hudde T, Minassian DC and Larkin DFP. Randomised controlled trial of corticosteroid regiments in endothelial corneal allograft rejection. *Br J Ophthalmol* 1999; 83:1348.
20. Hill JC. Immunosuppression in corneal transplantation. *Eye* 1995; 9(Pt 2): 247.
21. Hill JC. The use of cyclosporine in high-risk keratoplasty. *Am J Ophthalmol* 1989; 107: 506.
22. Hill JC. Systemic cyclosporine in high-risk keratoplasty: long-term results. *Eye* 1995; 9(Pt 4): 422.
23. Lam DS, Wong AK, Tham CC and Leung AT. The use of combined intravenous pulse methylprednisolone and oral cyclosporin A in the treatment of corneal graft rejection: a preliminary study. *Eye* 1998; 12(Pt 4): 615.
24. Young AL, Rao SK, Cheng LL, Wong AK, Leung AT and Lam DS. Combined intravenous pulse methylprednisolone and oral cyclosporine A in the treatment of corneal graft rejection: 5-year experience. *Eye* 2002; 16(3): 304.
25. Rumelt S, Bersudsky V, Blum-Hareuveni T and Rehany U. Systemic cyclosporin A in high failure risk, repeated corneal transplantation. *Br J Ophthalmol* 2002; 86(9): 988.
26. Sundmacher R and Reinhard T. Central corneolimbal transplantation under systemic ciclosporin A cover for severe limbal stem cell insufficiency. *Graefes Arch Clin Exp Ophthalmol* 1996; 234 Suppl 1: S122.

27. Algros MP, Angonin R, Delbosc B, Cahn JY and Kantelip B. Danger of systemic cyclosporine for corneal graft. *Cornea* 2002; 21(6): 613.
28. Vial T and Descotes J. Immunosuppressive drugs and cancer. *Toxicology* 2003; 185(3): 229.
29. Hunter PA, Wilhelmus KR, Rice NS and Jones BR. Cyclosporin A applied topically to the recipient eye inhibits corneal graft rejection. *Clin Exp Immunol* 1981; 45(1): 173.
30. Robert PY, Leconte V, Olive C, Ratsimbazafy V, Javerliat M and Adenis JP. Cyclosporin A eyedrops: manufacturing, toxicity, pharmacokinetics and indications in 2000. *J Fr Ophthalmol* 2001; 24(5): 527.
31. Pfau B, Kruse FE, Rohrschneider K, Zorn M, Fiehn W, Burk RO and Volcker HE. Comparison between local and systemic administration of cyclosporin A on the effective level in conjunctiva, aqueous humor and serum. *Ophthalmologe* 1995; 92(6): 833.
32. Field AJ and Gottsch JD. Persisting epithelial herpes simplex keratitis while on cyclosporin-A ointment. *Aust N Z J Ophthalmol* 1995; 23(4): 333.
33. Sloper CM, Powell RJ and Dua HS. Tacrolimus (FK506) in the management of high-risk corneal and limbal grafts. *Ophthalmology* 2001; 108(10): 1838.
34. Zamos DT and Tabin G. Tacrolimus (FK506) for high-risk corneal and limbal grafts. *Ophthalmology* 2002; 109(11): 1953.
35. Dua HS and Azuara-Blanco A. Allo-limbal transplantation in patients with limbal stem cell deficiency. *Br J Ophthalmol* 1999; 83(4): 414.
36. Reinhard T, Reis A, Kutkuhn B, Voiculescu A and Sundmacher R. Mycophenolate mofetil after penetrating high risk keratoplasty: a pilot study. *Klin Monatsbl Augenheilkd* 1999; 215(3): 201.
37. Reinhard T, Reis A, Bohringer D, Malinowski M, Voiculescu A, Heering P, Godehardt E and Sunmacher R. Systemic mycophenolate mofetil in comparison with systemic cyclosporin A in high-risk keratoplasty patients: 3 years' results of a randomized prospective clinical trial. *Graefes Arch Clin Exp Ophthalmol* 2001; 239(5): 367.
38. Reis A, Reinhard T, Voiculescu A, Kutkuhn B, Godehardt E, Spelsberg H, Althaus C and Sundmacher R. Mycophenolate mofetil versus cyclosporin A in high risk keratoplasty patients: a prospectively randomised clinical trial. *Br J Ophthalmol* 1999; 83(11): 1268.
39. Barraquer J. Immunosuppressive agents in penetrating keratoplasty. *Am J Ophthalmol* 1985; 100(1): 61.
40. Sudhir RR, Rao SK, Shanmugam MP and Padmanabhan P. Bilateral macular hemorrhage caused by azathioprine-induced aplastic anemia in a corneal graft recipient. *Cornea* 2002; 21(7): 712.
41. Berthoux F. Antibodies and immunomodulation. *Presse Med* 2001; 30(24, Pt 2): 41.
42. Lo A, Stratta RJ, Alloway RR, Egidi MF, Shokouh-Amiri MH, Grewal HP, Gaber LW and Gaber AO. Initial clinical experience with interleukin-2 receptor antagonist induction in combination with tacrolimus, mycophenolate mofetil and steroids in simultaneous kidney-pancreas transplantation. *Transpl Int* 2001; 14(6): 396.
43. Dick AD, Meyer P, James T, Forrester JV, Hale G, Waldmann H and Isaacs JD. Campath-1H therapy in refractory ocular inflammatory disease. *Br J Ophthalmol* 2000; 84(1):107.
44. Newman DK, Isaacs JD, Watson PG, Meyer PA, Hale G and Waldmann H. Prevention of immune-mediated corneal graft destruction with the anti-lymphocyte monoclonal antibody, CAMPATH-1H. *Eye* 1995; 9(Pt 5): 564.

45. Perico N and Remuzzi G. Prevention of transplant rejection: current treatment guidelines and future developments. *Drugs* 1997; 54(4): 533.
46. Fishbein TM, Florman S, Gondolesi G, Schiano T, LeLeiko N, Tschernia A and Kaufman S. Intestinal transplantation before and after the introduction of sirolimus. *Transplantation* 2002; 73(10): 1538.
47. Wu J and Zhou G. An experimental study of corneal allograft rejection with cytotoxin IL-2-PE40. *Chung Hua Yen Ko Tsa Chih* 1995; 31(5): 370.
48. Ponticelli C and Tarantino A. Promising new agents in the prevention of transplant rejection. *Drugs R D* 1999; 1(1): 55.

12

Transmission of Disease Through Corneal Transplantation

Introduction

At the time ophthalmology was emerging as a separate specialty in the early 19th century, the theoretical concept of replacing the scarified opaque cornea with a clear graft was converted into reality, as one of the earliest ophthalmic surgical procedures (see Chapter 1). However, the operation was not a success, and often disastrously so, not simply because the science of immunology, and the immunological principles of grafting, had not yet been discovered, but also because attempts to transplant animal corneas to humans, as was the practice in those early attempts at grafting, were frequently compounded by severe infection, due to primitive surgical techniques and lack of antisepsis and antibiotics. Now the most frequent form of solid organ transplant in humans (for review see [1]) corneal allograft is rarely complicated by infection. Nevertheless, infection is important as an initiator of graft rejection via induction of innate immunity (see Chapter 6) as well as a cause of graft failure.

The commonest form of infection of the graft is suture infection, leading to small intrastromal abscesses (see Chapter 3, Figure 3.3C). The source of infection is presumed to be acquired *de novo*, e.g. from airborne organisms, hand–eye contact, or a host reservoir of infection. However, it is possible that infection is transmitted via the donor and several examples of donor-related infection of the host graft, and even systemically of the host, have been described. This problem is not peculiar to cornea but has been recognised for many years as a risk with all types of solid organ graft [2]. In addition, many types of micro-organisms including viruses, aerobic bacteria, and fungi, as well as rarer infections such as trypanosoniasis and malaria have been transmitted via solid organ grafts. Prion disease, however, has only been transmitted iatrogenically via CNS or ocular tissue [2].

Bacterial and Fungal Disease

Only very rarely does transmission of bacterial infection via the graft threaten the life of the host (for review see [3]). Infection restricted to the corneal graft is more common and may take a variety of forms, including stromal keratitis, stitch abscess, crystalline keratopathy and endophthalmitis. Crystalline keratopathy, in which highly refractile stromal filaments develop in association with various micro-organisms including bacteria and fungi, is rare and the clinical features appear to be determined by the architecture of the cornea [4]. Some cases take the form of intrastromal biofilms [5].

The source of the infection can vary but has some relationship to time postgraft. Infections occurring in the early postoperative phase may be transmitted from the donor and in several large series of cases, there was a good correlation between positive culture of micro-organisms from the donor rim and culture of the sample taken from the grafted eye [6–8]. This applies to both bacterial and fungal infections.

In contrast, infections occurring at a later stage such as microbial keratitis or stitch abscess (see Chapter 3, Figure 3.3D) are more likely to have been introduced from nondonor sources, including the host [9]. Factors promoting infection include prolonged use of bandage contact lenses for non-healing epithelial defects, loose or broken sutures, adnexal/lid disease and intercurrent upper respiratory infections from the host.

Common micro-organisms involved in graft infection include pneumococcus and staphylococcus for stitch abscesses, while a range of virulent organisms, including *Pseudomonas aeruginosa*, have been causative for endophthalmitis. The reasons for failure of detection of donor associated micro-organisms is unclear. In fact, it is possible that the donor material is not infected but becomes contaminated during harvesting and processing, as was discovered in one small outbreak of pneumococcal endophthalmitis after keratoplasty [10]. The practice of culturing the donor button in tissue culture medium for some days prior to surgery has been associated with a higher rate of infection in some cases but may also help to identify donor buttons which are infected [11]. In some cases, infection has occurred when material was taken from donors who died of sepsis [12]. However, the recommendation not to accept corneas from donors who have died of sepsis (Eye Bank Association of America, 1996) has recently been challenged since prospective studies have not shown any greater increase in endophthalmitis using such material [11, 13–15]. In these studies it was observed that donor material from sepsis patients was less likely overall to be used for grafting since there was a higher rate of endothelial cell loss in donor buttons. Current techniques of preoperative donor button assessment may not be adequate for detecting infection.

Transmission of fungal infections from donor to host has also been documented as in the case *Candida albicans* [16]. Late infections (e.g. occurring in a clear graft some weeks after surgery) are almost certainly not donor related.

Virus Disease

Transmission of viral infection through donor corneal grafts is rare. The two best-known examples are hepatitis B and rabies.

Hepatitis B

The possibility of transmission of hepatitis B (and C) has been recognized for a long time and patients with known hepatitis B viraemia have been shown to express the surface antigen not only on vascularized structures within the eye but in the aqueous humour and on the corneal epithelium [17]. However, the first two cases of hepatitis B transmission via corneal graft were only reported in 1997 [18]. In both cases the serology and tissues from the donors were confirmed as positive when the infection became apparent in the recipients. Accordingly it is now standard practice to perform antibody screening tests of donors for hepatitis B (and C, although there is no reported case of hepatitis C transmission so far via the cornea). Due to the high false positive rates for these tests in screening assays, confirmatory testing of the donor is performed before the transplant is set aside, since there would be an excess wastage of donor material. A question has been raised regarding the need to exclude donor material from hepatitis B/C-positive donors since the risk of infection from such material has been estimated to be extremely low [19]. However, the current practice concerning serological testing in relation to donor tissue procurement in the USA has led to an excellent safety record in respect of viral infections [20].

Rabies

Transmission of rabies via donor cornea has a definitive history due to the likely fatal outcome. In the first reported case, the donor cornea of a forester who died of an undiagnosed rapidly developing neurological illness was transplanted to a 37-year-old woman with keratoconus. Four weeks post-transplant she developed neurological symptoms and after a further three weeks, she died. Rabies virus was recovered from both host and donor tissues [21]. Since then several other cases have been reported worldwide [3, 22–24]. Accordingly, it is standard practice to exclude all potential donors who have died from infectious, dementing neurological illness and in suspected cases, contacts of donor and host have been vaccinated against the virus [25].

Herpes viruses

One of the commonest indications for corneal grafting is herpetic stromal keratitis. Transmission of herpes virus to the host via the donor cornea has recently been reported in two cases who had no prior history of herpetic corneal disease [26]. One of the patients suffered primary graft failure and the second developed a persistent epithelial defect which also eventually ended in graft failure. Examination of the donor buttons revealed herpes virus particles which was confirmed by immunohistochemistry. The fellow donor button of one case developed endothelial necrosis while in culture. A similar suspected case, in which graft failure and endothelial necrosis was observed had been reported previously [27]. Direct evidence of herpes virions has been detected in corneal endothelial cells from a case of recurrent herpetic disease in a failed graft [28]. Transmission of latent herpetic virus which can replicate in both an anterograde and a retrograde manner from an infected donor to a naïve host has been shown to occur experimentally and infectivity appears to relate to the viral virulence rather than to host factors [29]. In humans, latent reactivation of herpetic infection in the donor graft is not uncommon. In one series, the rate of reactivation was 32% in cases undergoing rejection or a rejection episode, while in clear accepted grafts the rate was 6% [30]. Which of these two events (reactivation of infection and graft rejection) is cause or effect is not known but it is clear that induction of innate immunity by reactivation of infection is sufficient to initiate rejection (see Chapter 6). However, it is also possible, and probably more likely, that rejection of the graft is the initial event and that the use of intensive topical steroids to control the rejection episode induces overt herpetic infection. Thus prophylaxis with acyclovir in these cases greatly reduces recurrence of herpes [31, 32]. This has been tested experimentally in rabbits and shown to be a plausible mechanism [33].

Cytomegalovirus (CMV) and Epstein–Barr virus infections of the cornea are extremely rare. Experimentally the CMV promoter has been used to transfect donor endothelium with immunosuppressive cytokines such as IL-4 and IL-10 but the adenovirus and adeno-associated virus is more commonly used (see Chapter 10). In a large study of 110 corneas with active keratitis evaluated for various herpes viruses, no evidence for CMV or EBV was detected using sensitive PCR techniques. Corneal endothelial deposits are seen in patients with HIV and CMV retinitis but are not thought to be due to infective CMV but rather related to treatment with rifubatin [34–36]. Corneal epithelial infection with CMV has been described in a patient with AIDS [37].

HIV

Transmission of HIV by donor organ transplantation is also rare but has been reported for instance in cases of kidney transplantation [38]. No cases of HIV contracted through donor corneal transplantation have been recorded even when transplantation of a donor cornea from an HIV positive individual has inadvertently occurred [39]. Serologic testing for HIV is mandatory in most eye banks and additional sensitive testing using the p24 antigen has been suggested. This is particularly so since cadaveric serological testing has been shown not to be reliable for various viruses [40]. However, even where cases of donor corneas from p24+ individuals have been transplanted, HIV infection has not ensued [41]. As with prion disease (see below), the regulations with regard to HIV testing may be unnecessarily strict but difficult to change.

Prion Disease

Transmission of prion disease through corneal transplantation is famously reported. Prion diseases, otherwise known as the spongiform encephalopathies, include a range of mammalian diseases such as scrapie in sheep, bovine spongiform encephalopathy (BSE) in cattle, and Jacob-Creutzfeldt disease (CJD) and kuru in humans (for review see [42]). Most recently, in the wake of the BSE epidemic in the UK and other European countries, variant CJD (vCJD) has been attributed to cross-species infection via consumption of infected meat.

Prion disease is acquired through inoculation or ingestion of extracts of tissues, usually CNS tissues, from infected individuals. The term prion is derived from *pro*teinaceous and *in*fective. Prion proteins are a normal protease-sensitive constituent of CNS tissue, termed PrP^C, but become abnormal either by mutation, or functionally, by inducing large amounts of amyloid deposition in the presence of protease-resistant prion proteins (PrP^{SC} and PrP). In humans there are three forms of prion disease: sporadic CJD (sCJD), in which there is vacuolar degeneration with accumulation of PrP^{SC} and no PrP-associated amyloid plaque formation, inherited Gerstmann-type (GSS) disease, in which there is extensive amyloid plaque but in the presence of protease-sensitive PrP (ΔPrP), and the new variant vCJD with numerous protease-resistant PrP amyloid plaques. The pathogenesis of the disease is obscure but in essence it is believed that PrP^C becomes converted to PrP^{SC}/PrP by association with transmitted (ingested/inoculated) PrP^{SC}, and the increasing amounts of converted, protease resistant PrP^{SC} leads to the accumulation of amyloid material and brain degeneration. The result is a slow degenerative disease characterized by apoptosis of neuronal and glial cells, with progressive dementia, paralysis and finally death. The dominantly inherited form of the disease (GSS type disease) is believed to occur by spontaneous mutation of PrP^C to PrP^{SC} possibly in a stochastic manner. In humans the protein is encoded on Chromosome 20, and codon 129 of the *PRNP* (prion) gene is the site of mutation.

Transmission of CJD via corneal transplantation was first reported in 1974 in a woman who presented with ataxia 18 months after receiving a corneal graft from a man who died of "spongy" degeneration of the brain and was dead 8 months later [43]. Since then two further cases have been reported (reviewed in [44]). Experimental studies in guinea pigs demonstrated that this route of infection was truly mechanistic. In addition, further work revealed that the corneal epithelium of infected mink contains high levels transmissable particles, possibly associated with free nerve endings [45]. The iatrogenic form of prion disease is of the sCJD type. No case of vCJD transmitted via the cornea or other organ or blood transfusion, has been described despite concerns that some corneas have been cultured in fetal bovine serum.

Many questions remain. For instance it is not clear how PrP^{SC} invades the CNS. In vCJD and scrapie it has been shown that after oral ingestion or inoculation, PrP^{SC} replicates in the secondary lymphatic tissue where it colocalises with PrP^{C} on follicular dendritic cells [46]. Recent work suggests that it directly infects the nerves supplying splenic tissue and thus gains access to the CNS by retrograde spread along the axons. In addition, the risk of exposure to and infection by prion disease is not known. Recent epidemiological evidence indicates that there have been a few hundred cases of iatrogenic prion disease mostly from the use of cadaveric pituitary hormone preparations and dura mater grafts (rarely from ocular tissues) while around 110 cases of vCJD have been reported [44]. The size of the problem remains unknown but caution is advised. In the meantime, there is some possible good news in that recent studies in a murine model of scrapie have shown that a monoclonal antibody against PrP^{C} and PrP^{SC} can delay if not prevent development of the disease [47].

Conclusion

Transmission of disease through corneal transplantation is a rare but potentially life-threatening event. Adherence to guidelines for the retrieval, handling and storage of donor material currently ensures that the risk is low [48]. However, there is a corresponding impact on availability of donor material for transplantation.

References

1. Niederkorn JY. Mechanisms of corneal graft rejection: the sixth annual Thygeson lecture, presented at the ocular microbiology and immunology group meeting, October 21, 2000. *Cornea* 2001; 20(7): 675.
2. Gottesdiener KM. Transplanted infections: donor-to-host transmission with the allograft. *Ann Intern Med* 1989; 110(12): 1001.
3. O'Day DM. Diseases potentially transmitted through corneal transplantation. *Ophthalmology* 1989; 96(8): 1133; discussion 1137.
4. Butler TK *et al. In vitro* model of infectious crystalline keratopathy: tissue architecture determines pattern of microbial spread. *Invest Ophthalmol Vis Sci* 2001; 42(6): 1243.
5. Fulcher TP *et al.* Demonstration of biofilm in infectious crystalline keratopathy using ruthenium red and electron microscopy. *Ophthalmology* 2001; 108(6): 1088.

6. Aiello LP, Javitt JC and Canner JK. National outcomes of penetrating keratoplasty: risks of endophthalmitis and retinal detachment. *Arch Ophthalmol* 1993; 111(4): 509.
7. Pardos GJ and Gallagher MA. Microbial contamination of donor eyes: a retrospective study. *Arch Ophthalmol* 1982; 100(10): 1611.
8. Kloess PM *et al.* Bacterial and fungal endophthalmitis after penetrating keratoplasty. *Am J Ophthalmol* 1993; 115(3): 309.
9. Tseng SH and Ling KC. Late microbial keratitis after corneal transplantation. *Cornea* 1995; 14(6): 591.
10. Moore PJ *et al.* Pneumococcal endophthalmitis after corneal transplantation: control by modification of harvesting techniques. *Infect Control Hosp Epidemiol* 1989; 10(3): 102.
11. Armitage WJ and Easty DL. Factors influencing the suitability of organ-cultured corneas for transplantation. *Invest Ophthalmol Vis Sci* 1997; 38(1): 16.
12. Khodadoust AA and Franklin RM. Transfer of bacterial infections by donor cornea in penetrating keratoplasty. *Am J Ophthalmol* 1979; 87(2):130.
13. Spelsberg H *et al.* Organ-cultured corneal grafts from septic donors: a retrospective study. *Eye* 2002; 16(5): 622.
14. Robert PY *et al.* Internal and external contamination of donor corneas before in situ excision: bacterial risk factors in 93 donors. *Graefes Arch Clin Exp Ophthalmol* 2002; 240(4): 265.
15. Everts RJ *et al.* Corneoscleral rim cultures: lack of utility and implications for clinical decision-making and infection prevention in the care of patients undergoing corneal transplantation. *Cornea* 2001; 20(6): 586.
16. Sutphin JE *et al.* Donor-to-host transmission of *Candida albicans* after corneal transplantation. *Am J Ophthalmol* 2002; 134(1): 120.
17. Migden MR, Dennis WH and Clinch TE. Testing for hepatitis B surface antigen in processing donor tissue for penetrating keratoplasty. *Am J Ophthalmol* 1996; 122(3): 439.
18. Hoft RH *et al.* Clinical evidence for hepatitis B transmission resulting from corneal transplantation. *Cornea* 1997; 16(2): 132.
19. Sengler U *et al.* Testing of corneoscleral discs and their culture media of seropositive donors for hepatitis B and C virus genomes. *Graefes Arch Clin Exp Ophthalmol* 2001; 239(10): 783.
20. Glasser DB. Serologic testing of cornea donors. *Cornea* 1998; 17(2): 123.
21. Houff SA *et al.* Human-to-human transmission of rabies virus by corneal transplant. *N Engl J Med* 1979; 300(11): 603.
22. Gandhi SS, Lamberts DW and Perry HD . Donor to host transmission of disease via corneal transplantation. *Surv Ophthalmol* 1981; 25(5): 306.
23. Javadi MA *et al.* Transmission of rabies by corneal graft. *Cornea* 1996; 15(4): 431.
24. Gode GR and Bhide NK. Two rabies deaths after corneal grafts from one donor. *Lancet* 1988; 2(8614): 791.
25. Anderson LJ *et al.* Nosocomial rabies: investigation of contacts of human rabies cases associated with a corneal transplant. *Am J Pub Health* 1984; 74(4): 370.
26. Biswas S *et al.* Graft failure in human donor corneas due to transmission of herpes simplex virus. *Br J Ophthalmol* 2000; 84(7): 701.
27. Cleator GM *et al.* Corneal donor infection by herpes simplex virus: herpes simplex virus DNA in donor corneas. *Cornea* 1994; 13(4): 294.

28. Holbach LM, Asano N and Naumann GO. Infection of the corneal endothelium in herpes simplex keratitis. *Am J Ophthalmol* 1998; 126(4): 592.
29. Zheng X *et al.* HSV-1 migration in latently infected and naive rabbits after penetrating keratoplasty. *Invest Ophthalmol Vis Sci* 1999; 40(11): 2490.
30. Cobo LM *et al.* Prognosis and management of corneal transplantation for herpetic keratitis. *Arch Ophthalmol* 1980; 98(10): 1755.
31. Ficker LA *et al.* The changing management and improved prognosis for corneal grafting in herpes simplex keratitis. *Ophthalmology* 1989; 96(11): 1587.
32. Simon AL and Pavan-Langston D. Long-term oral acyclovir therapy: effect on recurrent infectious herpes simplex keratitis in patients with and without grafts. *Ophthalmology* 1996; 103(9): 1399; discussion 1404.
33. Beyer CF *et al.* Penetrating keratoplasty in rabbits induces latent HSV-1 reactivation when corticosteroids are used. *Curr Eye Res* 1989; 8(12): 1323.
34. Holland SP *et al.* Corneal endothelial deposits in patients with HIV infection or AIDS: epidemiologic evidence of the contribution of rifabutin. *Can J Ophthalmol* 1999; 34(4): 204.
35. Inoue T *et al.* Corneal infiltration and CMV retinitis in a patient with AIDS. *Cornea* 1998; 17(4): 441.
36. Miedziak AI, Rapuano CJ and Goldman S. Corneal endothelial precipitates in HIV- and CMV-positive patients without concomitant ocular disease. *Eye* 1998; 12 (Pt 4): 743.
37. Wilhelmus KR *et al.* Cytomegalovirus keratitis in acquired immunodeficiency syndrome. *Arch Ophthalmol* 1996; 114(7): 869.
38. Schwarz A *et al.* Human immunodeficiency virus transmission by organ donation: outcome in cornea and kidney recipients. *Transplantation* 1987; 44(1): 21.
39. Caron MJ and Wilson R. Review of the risk of HIV infection through corneal transplantation in the United States. *J Am Optom Assoc* 1994; 65(3): 173.
40. Heim A *et al.* Evaluation of serological screening of cadaveric sera for donor selection for cornea transplantation. *J Med Virol* 1999; 58(3): 291.
41. Chung CW *et al.* Human immunodeficiency virus p24 antigen testing in cornea donors. *Cornea* 2001; 20(3): 277.
42. DeArmond SJ and Bouzamondo E. Fundamentals of prion biology and diseases. *Toxicology* 2002; 181–182: 9.
43. Duffy P *et al.* Letter: Possible person-to-person transmission of Creutzfeldt–Jakob disease. *N Engl J Med* 1974; 290(12): 692.
44. Pedersen NS and Smith E. Prion diseases: epidemiology in man. *Apmis* 2002; 110(1): 14.
45. Marsh RF and Hanson RP. Transmissible mink encephalopathy: infectivity of corneal epithelium. *Science* 1975; 187(4177): 656.
46. Brown KL *et al.* Scrapie replication in lymphoid tissues depends on prion protein-expressing follicular dendritic cells. *Nat Med* 1999; 5(11): 1308.
47. White AR *et al.* Monoclonal antibodies inhibit prion replication and delay the development of prion disease. *Nature* 2003; 422(6927): 80.
48. Allan B and Tuft S. Transmission of Creutzfeldt–Jakob disease in corneal grafts. *Br Med J* 1997; 315(7122): 1553.

13

Artificial Corneas

Introduction

The significant advances towards successful penetrating keratoplasty (PK) during the last half century are well recognized, but many problems remain. Long term graft acceptance declines with time, and certain groups of patients with severely scarified corneas particularly fail to do well with PK. Alternative approaches have been adopted and, since the original suggestion by Gillaume Pellier de Quengsy (see Chapter 1), many attempts to fashion an artificial cornea have been made (for review see [1]). This has led to several recent developments in artificial corneas or keratoprostheses (KPro) and the field is rich with ideas from biomaterials experts. However, as a solution to a global problem, KPro is unlikely to provide an answer to the large amount of corneal scarring disease which accounts for a significant level of world blindness especially from diseases such as trachoma and nutritional deficiency despite interest from several groups worldwide. Little more than 5000 KPros in total have been inserted compared to the large number of PKs performed annually (>40 000 in the US alone) [1].

The main reason for this situation is that developments in prosthetic corneas, unlike artificial lenses or hip joints, face many obstacles mostly due to complications, early and late. Difficulties arise in ensuring biocompatibility of the artificial material, which as a foreign material drives chronic inflammation, prevents good healing and leads to the inevitable complications of wound leak, hypotony, retinal detachment and infection. Even if some degree of biocompatibility is achieved, retroprosthesis membranes form, derived in part from epithelial downgrowths. In addition, the constant need for prolonged, careful postoperative care which apply even more to KPro than to PK (see Chapter 2) have prevented KPros from wider availability.

The most significant advances in KPro came from developments in plastics, particularly polymethylmethacrylate, which were seen serendipitously during World War II, to be relatively inert when lodged in ocular tissues. However, most workers in this field have developed an interest in one or other particular KPro model due mainly to the fact that experience is limited in each centre to small numbers of cases in which it would be almost ethically impossible to conduct a controlled trial comparing the various models.

Biomaterials

The most commonly used material for manufacture of KPros has been polymethylmethacrylate (PMMA). Some are made entirely of PMMA (the collar stud variety; see below) while others are a composite of various materials of which the central optic cylinder is PMMA and the surrounding skirt may be composed of a variety of polymers which have been perforated to make them more porous and therefore adherent to the tissues (Figure 13.1). These include: perforated grids of PMMA, nylon, ceramics, Teflon, Proplast, (Vitek Inc, Houston,TX, USA), polytetrafluoroethylene and polyurethane. Hydrogels, including collagen gels with various additions such as chondroitin sulphate, have also been used. A three-piece KPro incorporating PMMA and two other polymers, e.g. a polyurethane and polypropylene haptics, have also been introduced recently [2] and found in short term studies to be stable in humans. Poly(2-hydroxyethyl methacrylate)(PHEMA) has been the focus of intense interest in this field since it is well tolerated by biological tissues, e.g. intraocular and contact lenses, but there is a tendency for them to calcify if they are prepared as sponges.

Finally the Aachen KPro is prepared entirely from silicone and is used as a temporary prosthesis, sutured to the cornea, as an aid to vitreoretinal surgery in patients requiring multiple, simultaneous surgical procedures (see Chapter 2).

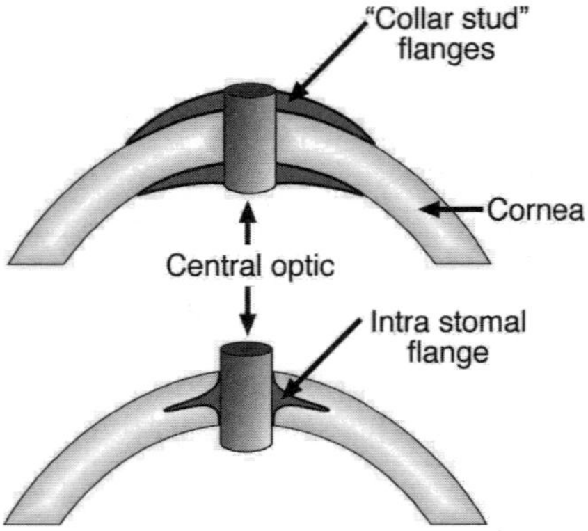

Figure 13.1 Diagrams of the two main types of keratoprosthesis.

Indications for KPro

Many ocular surface disorders are potentially treatable with KPro. These include corneal opacification due to chemical burns, fibrotic surface disease such as ocular cicatricial pemphigoid, Stevens–Johnson syndrome, and recurrent graft failure. Some of these conditions respond better to the presence of the KPro than others and this depends on whether there is an underlying ongoing inflammation. The most successful results have been obtained in recurrent graft failures.

Contraindications for KPro include disorders in which there is active inflammatory or infective corneal disease, conditions where there is extensive thinning of the corneal surface especially towards the periphery and cases where imaging or other functional preoperative tests have revealed disease of the posterior segment. Assessment using ultrasound biomicroscopy may also provide information on the suitability of the case by revealing structural damage to the anterior segment which may preclude the use of a KPro.

Types of Keratoprosthesis

There are two basic designs of KPro in use (Figure 13.1): the collar stud design, in which the central optical stem connects two plates which fit over the edge of the cornea and are sewn into place like a PK; and the skirt type of KPro, in which the central optical stem is attached to a thin skirt which is inserted into the cornea like a lamellar graft and overlaid with a mucous membrane graft. The latter type is more commonly used. Modifications of these models are in use. The optical portion of the device is usually prepared from polymethylmethacrylate (PMMA) or a derivative thereof, since this is a completely clear and inert material as used in many types of intraocular lens. The flanges or skirts have been prepared from other materials to promote biocompatibility, sometimes with pores to promote ingrowth of host keratocytes. Difficulties arise mostly in relation to the peripheral skirt which may not integrate well with the cornea. Many attempts to improve biointegration, as it is known, have been made by using modified types of PMMA such as HPMMA, a more hydrophilic version of the plastic.

The Dohlmann–Doane KPro

This device is an all PMMA KPro of the collar stud variety and is of two types, a short version for "wet" eyes and a longer device with an additional through-the-lid component for very dry eyes. Most KPros are designed on a similar model composed of a central tubular stem containing the optic which traverses a central 2–3 mm diameter trephined defect in the cornea and a skirt which inserts into the surrounding corneal tissue (Figure 13.1). Usually the KPro is held in place with an overlapping conjunctival flap or with lid skin which initially covers the central optic until full healing takes place. Opening of the flap is performed after about two months.

Lensectomy, iridectomy and vitrectomy are performed as necessary (see Chapter 2) and postoperatively antibiotics, and high dose immunosuppression with steroids and other regimens, are required to prevent inflammation particularly uveitis which can be difficult to evaluate.

A retrospective analysis of the results of the use of this KPro in a series of 63 patients has shown good overall benefit in 55 cases, one spontaneous extrusion and 10 cases which did not respond visually. Patients whose indication for KPro was repeated graft failure seemed to have the best prognosis [3].

The Strampelli osteo-odonto KPro

During the 1960s and early 70s Strampelli pioneered a novel approach to resolving the problem of biointegration [4]. After some research in primates which confirmed the feasability of the technique [5, 6], he developed an osteo-odonto KPro. Using a fragment of the patient's dental bone taken from the jaw as a support for the central lenticular optic, he first embedded the prosthesis in an eyelid/cheek pouch for several weeks to ensure that it became infiltrated with fibroblasts, and developed attachments and firm adhesions to the patient's connective tissue [7]. Then he removed the osteo-odonto prosthesis and inserted it into a layer of buccal mucosa that had been used to cover a trephined defect in the cornea. He reported some success with this procedure with long term stability in some cases.

The procedure was further developed by Falcinelli in the last decade of the 20th century [8] and later by Pintucci *et al.* using a Dacron support instead of autologous bone [9, 10]. In recent years this model has been introduced by CS Liu into the UK [11, 12]. Continued research in this area is aimed at developing better plastic which will allow integration with keratocytes and prevent epithelial downgrowth which is the major cause of failure and extrusion of these KPros[11]. In addition, the small visual field achieved with the cylindrical optic can be improved using modified lens designs [13]. Despite the prolonged surgery and the expensive process of visual rehabilitation in these cases, the advances achieved in these often complex and difficult cases has proved to be cost-effective [14].

The Chirilla KPro (Alphcor)

The AlphaCor KPro is also a core-and-skirt device but composed of a hydrogel synthetic cornea. A white porous skirt surrounds the central optical core and is intended to permit integration with the corneal tissue preventing epithelial downgrowth. The device is inserted in a two-stage procedure in which the recipient cornea is first dissected to create an intrastromal pocket of 7 mm diameter. A central 3 mm of the posterior lamellae of the cornea is removed using a disposable trephine and the device inserted into the intrastromal pocket which is then sutured. A conjunctival flap is then prepared to cover the anterior surface of the cornea.

The main advantage of the Alphcor is that if complications such as tissue necrosis and corneal melts occur, the KPro is reversible and a standard penetrating keratoplasty (PK) can be performed [15] and as such it has a good safety record so far [16]. To date 49 devices have been implanted into 45 eyes, in which 80% had a 1-year survival (Crawford *et al.*, personal communication). The main associated cause of tissue melt is in cases of herpes simplex eye disease where survival of the device is poor. In addition, experience in severe dry eye disease has not been widely reported.

Complications of KPros

The major complications of KPros are tissue necrosis around the implant which can lead to wound leak, endophthalmitis and retinal detachment.

Attempts to resuture the device can be made using additional material such as fascia lata. However, most of these complications are difficult to manage and have a poor prognosis. Glaucoma is also a complication and may require to be managed prophylactically with a valve device. Retroprosthesis membranes can be treated with laser therapy. As indicated in a recent editorial, no current prosthesis permits a covering of host epithelium and until this difficulty can be overcome, the problem of epithelial downgrowth and extrusion cannot be resolved [17].

Human Corneal Functional Equivalents

The problem of biointegration of plastic materials with biological tissues has prevented widespread use of KPros and limited their success overall. Accordingly, attempts have been made to develop polymeric synthetic corneas which are seeded with cells and support an endothelial monolayer [18]. Griffith *et al.* reported on such a model which appeared to retain optical and functional qualities of a normal cornea. The structure was based on a collagen gel matrix, and epithelial and endothelial cells were seeded on the appropriate surfaces. Further work has been performed using collagen cross-linkers to produce a hybrid biosynthetic tissue replacement to enhance the toughness of the gel and render it suitable for suturing to the cornea [18] (Figure 13.2). Initial experiments using this material as lamellar grafts in rabbits and minipigs have been performed with good results and minimal or no inflammation, as shown by the histology (Figure 13.3A–C) (Griffiths, personal communication).

Other approaches have been designed such as using donor corneal stroma, denuded of Descemet's membrane as a template for seeding endothelial cells [19]. Both human or porcine adult corneal endothelial cells were used and maintained in monolayer cultures before seeding. Between 150 000 and 700 000 cells seeded onto recipient corneas, followed by gentle centrifugation to improve attachment, allowed maximal final numeric cell densities of 3450/mm^2 and 1850/ for pig and human lines, respectively. The most effective method for denuding the donor cornea of its own endothelium was freezing-and-thawing. The newly established endothelial monolayer remained stable for up to 20 days in organ culture and appeared to function well as a fluid pump since the stroma reduced thickness to near physiological levels. More recently, immortalized endothelial cell lines have been used to cover denuded murine cornea and tested *in vivo*, with some encouraging results [20].

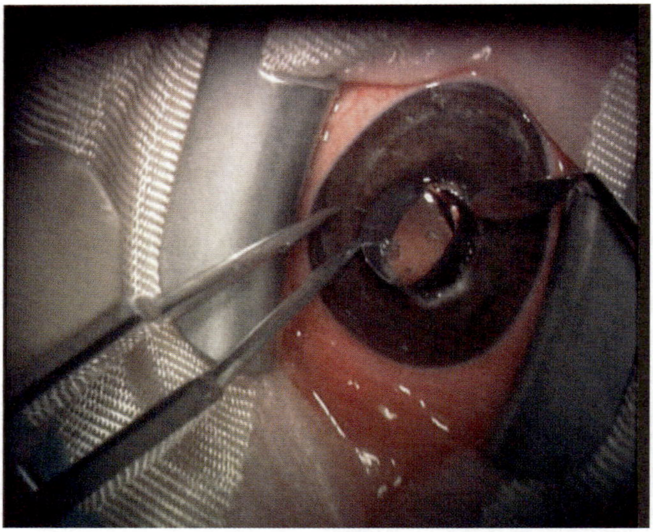

Figure 13.2 Synthetic, polymeric artificial cornea being implanted into minipig eye. (*Courtesy M. Griffith.*)

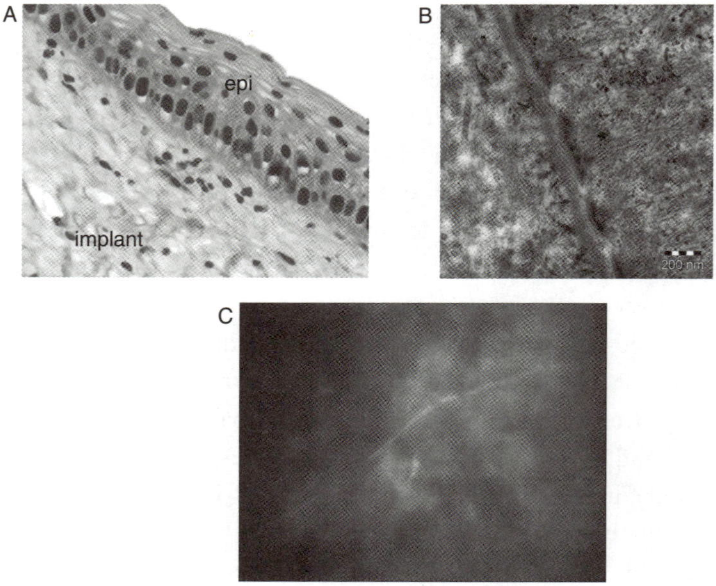

Figure 13.3 Histology of synthetic cornea six weeks postoperatively in minipig eye. Epithelial cell regrowth on implant (**A**); showing establishment of hemidesmosomes in re-established basement membrane (**B**); (**C**) subepithelial nerve within polymeric implant. (*Courtesy M. Griffith.*)

Conclusion

While considerable advances have been made in developments of KPros, and some patients have benefited greatly from their use, there are still challenges to be overcome. In essence, the main problem is the tendency of foreign material to be extruded due to the fact that it induces either a chronic inflammation in the tissue, with melting and necrosis of the leucomatous cornea or it tends to become walled off within a capsule formed by epithelial downgrowth and a retroprosthesis membrane. Patients with an underlying inflammatory condition such as Stevens–Johnson syndrome and the long term effects of chemical burns tend to do less well than those with scleralized corneas from repeated rejections of corneal grafts, unless the reason for graft failure is inflammatory disease such as herpetic eye disease.

References

1. Dohlman C and Power WJ *Keratoprosthesis,* 2nd ed., *Principles and Practice of Ophthalmology*, eds. Albert DM and Jakobiec FA, Vol. 2. W.B. Saunders, Philadelphia, 2000; 1069.
2. Kim MK *et al.* Seoul-type keratoprosthesis: preliminary results of the first 7 human cases. *Arch Ophthalmol* 2002; 120(6): 761.
3. Yaghouti F *et al.* Keratoprosthesis: preoperative prognostic categories. *Cornea* 2001; 20(1): 19.
4. Strampelli B. Kertoprosthesis with osteodontal tissue. *Am J Ophthalmol* 1963; 89: 1029.
5. Strampelli B and Restivo Manfridi ML. Histological study of autografts of dental roots in the eyelid of Macacus rhesus. II. *Ann Ottalmol Clin Ocul* 1969; 95(9): 709.
6. Strampelli B and Restivo-Manfridi ML. Histological study of autografts of dental root in the eyelid of Macacus rhesus. I. *Ann Ottalmol Clin Ocul* 1967; 93(12): 1437.
7. Strampelli B. Osteo-odonto keratoprosthesis. *Ber Zusammenkunft Dtsch Ophthalmol Ges* 1972; 71: 322.
8. Falcinelli GC *et al.* Detection of glaucomatous damage in patients with osteo-odontokeratoprosthesis. *Br J Ophthalmol* 1995; 79(2): 129.
9. Pintucci S *et al.* The Dacron felt colonizable keratoprosthesis: after 15 years. *Eur J Ophthalmol* 1996; 6(2): 125.
10. Pintucci S *et al.* Influence of dacron tissue thickness on the performance of the Pintucci biointegrable keratoprosthesis: an *in vitro* and *in vivo* study. *Cornea* 2001; 20(6): 647.
11. Sandeman SR *et al.* Novel materials to enhance keratoprosthesis integration. *Br J Ophthalmol* 2000; 84(6): 640.
12. Liu C *et al.* Osteon-odonto-keratoprosthesis surgery. *Br J Ophthalmol* 1999; 83(1): 127.
13. Hull CC *et al.* Optical cylinder designs to increase the field of vision in the osteo-odonto-keratoprosthesis. *Graefes Arch Clin Exp Ophthalmol* 2000; 238(12): 1002.
14. Geerling G *et al.* Costs and gains of complex procedures to rehabilitate end stage ocular surface disease. *Br J Ophthalmol* 2002; 86(11): 1220.

15. Hicks CR *et al.* Outcomes of implantation of an artificial cornea, AlphaCor: effects of prior ocular herpes simplex infection. *Cornea* 2002; 21(7): 685.
16. Crawford GJ *et al.* The Chirila keratoprosthesis: phase I human clinical trial. *Ophthalmology* 2002; 109(5): 883.
17. Allan B. Artificial corneas. *Br Med J* 1999; 318(7187): 821.
18. Griffith M *et al.* Artificial human corneas: scaffolds for transplantation and host regeneration. *Cornea* 2002; 21(7 Suppl): S54.
19. Engelmann K, Drexler D and Bohnke M. Transplantation of adult human or porcine corneal endothelial cells onto human recipients in vitro. Part I: Cell culturing and transplantation procedure. *Cornea* 1999; 18(2): 199.
20. Joo CK *et al.* Repopulation of denuded murine Descemet's membrane with life-extended murine corneal endothelial cells as a model for corneal cell transplantation. *Graefes Arch Clin Exp Ophthalmol* 2000; 238(2): 174.

Index